Keto for Beginners

Diana Lor & Anna Watson

Copyright 2018 by Diana Lor & Anna Watson
All rights reserved.

The following Book is reproduced below with the goal of providing information that is as accurate and reliable as possible. Regardless, purchasing this Book can be seen as consent to the fact that both the publisher and the author of this book are in no way experts on the topics discussed within and that any recommendations or suggestions that are made herein are for entertainment purposes only. Professionals should be consulted as needed prior to undertaking any of the action endorsed herein.

This declaration is deemed fair and valid by both the American Bar Association and the Committee of Publishers Association and is legally binding throughout the United States.

Furthermore, the transmission, duplication or reproduction of any of the following work including specific information will be considered an illegal act irrespective of if it is done electronically or in print. This extends to creating a secondary or tertiary copy of the work or a recorded copy and is only allowed with express written consent from the Publisher. All additional right reserved.

The information in the following pages is broadly considered to be a truthful and accurate account of facts and as such any inattention, use or misuse of the information in question by the reader will render any resulting actions solely under their purview. There are no scenarios in which the publisher or the original author of this work can be in any fashion deemed liable for any hardship or damages that may befall them after undertaking information described herein.

Additionally, the information in the following pages is intended only for informational purposes and should thus be thought of as universal. As befitting its nature, it is presented without assurance regarding its prolonged validity or interim quality. Trademarks that are mentioned are done without written consent and can in no way be considered an endorsement from the trademark holder.

Table of Contents

Introduction 1

What Is Keto? 3

   Is Keto Diet the Right Option? 5

   Different Types of Keto Diets 7

      The Standard Keto Diet 7

      The Targeted Keto Diet 8

      The High-Protein Keto Diet 9

      The Cyclical Keto Diet 10

   Research 12

   Comparison with Other High-Efficiency Dietary Plans 13

      Atkins Diet 13

      The Paleo Diet 14

      Intermittent Fasting 15

   Why You Should Go with the Keto Diet 15

   Potential Disadvantages 16

   Myths Concerning the Keto Diet 18

      Keto Diet is high in protein. 18

Any type of fat is admissible. 19

The brain is not able to function properly without carbs. 20

It is a long-term solution. 20

Getting Started 22

Common Mistakes People Make in Keto Diet ... 22

Using the Keto Diet as a Quick Fix 23

Being Afraid of Fats 23

Eating Too Much Protein 24

Not Taking Enough Water 24

Not Getting the Right Amount of Sleep 25

Looking at the Scale 25

Key Steps in Getting Started with Keto 26

You will not eat… 27

You can eat… 27

Calculating the Level of Carbs 28

Make the Environment Open to the Keto Diet .. 29

Prepare for the Keto Flu 30

Be Mindful of the Amounts of Food That You Are Eating 30

Keto Diet Do's and Don'ts 31

    The Do's 31

    The Don'ts.. 38

How The Keto Diet Works 43

Fats, Carbs, and Proteins 46

The Importance of Fat When It Comes to the Keto Diet 46

Calorie Intake Is Significant. 47

How to Increase Fat Intake?.................................... 48

Sources of Healthy Fats 48

Daily Protein Requirements.................................... 49

Good and Bad Foods and Drinks to Consume on Keto... 51

    Meat.. 51

    Eggs 52

    Natural Fat and High-Fat Sauces 52

    Fish and Seafood.. 52

    Vegetables That Are Grown Above Ground .. 53

    Nuts 53

    High-Fat Dairy 54

    Coffee 54

    Tea... 54

- Bone Broth 55
- Grains 55

Thoughts on Good vs. Bad Carbs 55

Bad Carbs While on the Keto Diet (Sugars and Starch) 57

Condiments, Herbs, and Spices 57

Alcohol and the Keto Diet..................................... 58

Health Benefits & Possible Side Effects of Keto. 60

- Health Benefits.. 60
  - Low-carb diets kill appetite. 60
  - Bigger proportions of the fat lost are from the abdominal space.. 61
  - Low Blood Sugar 62
  - Weight Loss.. 62
  - Brain Function 64
  - Endurance Performance..................................... 66
  - Stable Levels of Energy 67
  - Migraine Treatment 69
  - Low-carb diets are therapeutic for brain disorders. 69
  - Better Sleep Patterns 70

- Reduction of Inflammation Issues/Marks 71
- Healthier Liver 71
- Mood Stabilization for Autism and Bipolar Disorders 72
- It Is Easier to Fast 73
- Irritable Bowel Syndrome 73
- Anti-Aging 74
- Cancer 75
- Acne 76

Potential Side Effects of the Keto Diet 76
- Inflammation 77
- Bad Breath 78
- Keto Rash 79
- Urine 80
- The Keto Flu 80
- Constipation 82
- Yo-Yo Dieting 83
- Kidney and Heart Damage 83
- Diarrhea 84
- Muscle Cramps 85
- Nutritional Problems 85

  Sleeping Problems 86

Pregnancy and Ketosis 87

  Natural Scenarios of Ketosis in Women Who Are Pregnant 88

  Ketosis During the Late Stage of Pregnancy .. 89

  The Controversy When It Comes to the Keto Diet 89

  The Low-Carb States and Pregnancy 90

  Precautions 91

Common Mistakes People Make on Keto 94

  #1 – The Wrong Fats 95

  #2 – Eating Too Much Protein 96

  #3 – Too Little Water 97

  #4 – Focusing on the Food Alone 99

  #5 – Obsessing Over Weight 100

Recipes & Meal Plans 102

  How Do Meal Plans Work? 106

  How to Find the Daily Need? 107

Snack Recipes for the Keto Diet 109

Breakfast Recipes 121

Lunch Recipes 133

Dinner Recipes...145

Introduction

The Ketogenic diet is a low-carb, high-fat diet with a lot of similarities shared with the Atkins and Low-Carb diet. It entails reducing the intake of carbohydrates and replacing them with foods rich in fat. That elimination of carbohydrates for the daily diet and the intake of natural fats is what places the body within a metabolic state known as Ketosis. The body becomes efficient in burning fat that is taken for the purpose of producing energy. It turns the fat to ketones within the liver, which then allows for the supply of energy to the brain. Ketogenic diets allow for reductions in the levels of blood sugar and insulin as well, which makes for good health benefits.

Nutritional Ketosis happens when the body burns fat rather than sugar in order to come up with fuel. It is also a way for you to improve your health significantly—and it entails eating a diet with the carb having the lowest percentage, protein at a moderate level, and fat at the highest level within your diet. This may then seem counter-intuitive, as many have been taught that the best thing is to restrict dietary fat and to consume big portions of carbohydrates, particularly whole grains. However, the truth, as proven by a number of medical studies, is that eating more fat and a lesser amount of carbohydrates is better for a wide range of health issues. It will assist with weight loss, improvement of mental focus, and an increase in levels of energy — all the while stabilizing the levels of blood sugar and balancing hormones.

This short book is an introduction to the Ketogenic diet and will illustrate what it is and how it affects the body — not to mention potential health benefits and meal plans. Unlike the other traditional guides to the Ketogenic process, it does not focus on calories or the manipulation of macros or following particular rules to the latter. Instead, it allows freedom and flexibility to do what feels like the appropriate thing to benefit your health. With the recipes and strategies in this book, it will become possible for you to be able to end unhealthy relationships with food and to create restrictions through appropriate nutritional practices. In doing so, you can attain the health and weight you aspire.

Chapter 1

WHAT IS KETO?

The Ketogenic diet first became popular during the 20s as a treatment for diabetes and epilepsy. Generally, the limit for carbs in the Keto diet is set at no more than 50 grams every day, which would be equal to a cup of what rice or a bagel has. However, the dietary guidelines laid out by the U.S. Department of Agriculture recommend the consumption of between 225 and 325 grams of carbohydrates every day. During the Keto diet, the body goes into a state of starvation—hence, it taps the fat stores for fuel. Numerous studies suggest the high-fat and low-carb diet would result in dull hunger, but it would promote weight loss. It also helps in preventing age-related illnesses. As such, an increasing number of health enthusiasts from various online platforms are supporting the Keto diet.

The Keto diet reorganizes the formation of the food pyramid. It cuts on the carbs and sets a limit between

20 and 50 grams every day—depending on one's medical history and insulin sensitivity. In this diet, healthy fats would have to account for about 70 percent of the daily calories taken by the individual, and protein should only account for 25 percent. The current statistics show that most people consume half of their calories from carbs, 15% from protein intake, and 30 % from fat.

During the creation of energy, the human body initiates the breakdown of carbs into glucose, which is broken down into constituents for glycogen in the liver and energy for the body. In the absence of carbohydrates, the body initiates its secondary protocol by using up the glucose reserves and breaking down the stored fat into fatty acids. When the acids reach the liver, they are subsequently converted into an organic substance known as ketones. The brain along with other organs then feed on the ketones in a process referred to as Ketosis—thus giving birth to this dietary process. To help maintain this state Keto dieters eat a lot of healthy fats.

Is Keto Diet the Right Option?

The body sends signals to the brain at every moment of the day on what it requires. If you do not pay attention to these signals, you might keep doing things leading to discontentment concerning the state of your health. The good news is that it is not a must for you to sit on a meditation pillow for hours in order to know what the body requires. For a lot of people, the increase of fat intake and lowering the levels of carb consumption along with some self-care would be the starting point needed to give the body exactly what it needs.

If you are wondering whether the body really wants or needs more fat, there are some signs that you may refer to. If you recognize some of the following symptoms, then it could be a sign you need additional healthy fats within your diet.

- ➢ You experience weight gain, sluggishness, headaches, and random symptoms—thus making the day challenging.
- ➢ You have tried all eating styles, but none of them assists in making you feel good or looking great.

- You need pick-me-ups in the afternoon to keep your brain working.
- Your hormones are all over the place, and you have frequent mood swings.
- You can eat even thirty minutes after you have had a meal.
- You become allergic or sensitive to foods that you never used to have a reaction to.
- After thirty minutes of having a meal, you experience a lot of sleepiness to the point you are not effective unless you have had a nap.
- You have moments of emotional highs and lows and have a hard time understanding what created the imbalance or remembering that it happened in the first place.

If you are feeling or have felt any of the symptoms that were stated, then the Keto diet may just be the thing to assist you to have a fuller and more effective lifestyle.

Different Types of Keto Diets

The Standard Keto Diet

The Standard Keto Diet (SKD) is the most common type of Keto diet, and experts alternatively refer to it as the Very Low Carb Keto Diet (VLCKD).

In essence, the SKD is low on carbs, utilizes moderate amounts of protein, and have high levels of fat—specifically 5% carbs, 20% protein, and a whopping 75% fats. For an average person, these proportions translate to a 30-gram daily intake of carbs.

Generally, this type of diet veers away from starches, excessive sugar, fruits, and other high-carb foods. Instead, it focuses on those that are low in carbs such as seeds, nuts, low-carb veggies, and high-fat dairy products.

This type of Keto diet is ideal for people who aim to have a weight drop within a short period of time while only being required of light exercises/workout routines such as cycling, walking, light weightlifting, and yoga. It is fairly simple to follow, and it allows you to take your carbs whenever you feel like you need them.

However, like everything else in the world, the Standard keto diet is not meant for everyone — among them are pregnant women, people with a history of kidney stones, and those with diabetes.

The Targeted Keto Diet

The Targeted Keto Diet (TKD) involves taking up carbs before your workouts — preferably within an hour prior. During this time, you will be able to suffice your daily carb goal of 30 grams.

In essence, the targeted keto diet is just a modified version of the standard diet — with the only difference being the specified period for taking up your carbs.

Generally, the targeted diet veers away and focuses on the same types of foods as previously mentioned for the standard diet. However, the added modification aims to provide the necessary nutrients (which are found in carb-rich foods) to serve as "fuel" for an efficient performance during workouts or exercises — especially those that are relatively intense—while at the same time making sure that the process of Ketosis is not disturbed for extended periods.

For this type of Keto diet, it is preferred for you to choose carbs that are quite easy to digest like white rice or white bread, so as to minimize its impact to Ketosis while still providing carbs when you need it the most, i.e. for workouts.

The targeted diet is ideal for people who are undergoing intensive activities with the goal of building up muscles. Likewise, it is also good for people who are only starting in working out and are not yet ready to undergo a more complex type of diet.

The High-Protein Keto Diet

The High-Protein Keto Diet is another modified version of the standard diet, except that it involves taking up more protein so that the proportion of fat is slightly reduced as a result. The protein ratio is now set at 35%, the fat ratio is lowered to 60%, while the carbs remain at 5%—thus essentially still following the basic idea of a Ketogenic diet.

Generally, this type of diet veers away from high-carb foods as well as overly fatty dishes. Instead, it focuses on those that are high in protein such as dairy, meat, nuts, fish and seeds.

This type of Keto diet is ideal for bodybuilders or other people who need to up their protein intake so as to maintain their muscle mass. This can also be beneficial to elderly people who want to achieve the benefits of a Keto diet but at the same time prevent muscle breakdown. Furthermore, this is ideal for people who show signs of protein deficiency, such as thinning hair and muscle loss.

However, experts advise caution for people who have issues with their kidneys so as to avoid unnecessary waste build-up in the blood. Also, too much protein in a Keto diet is discouraged, as it can significantly decrease the amount of ketones (a substance needed for Ketosis) in one's blood — thus making it important for people to stick to the prescribed proportions as much as possible.

The Cyclical Keto Diet

The Cyclical Keto Diet (CKD), alternatively referred to as carb-cycling, is a low-carb diet added with intermittent "carb refeeding days" for when its users need to undergo highly intensive activities.

In essence, the cyclical diet is just a hybrid version of the standard diet—with the main difference having a provision for high-carb consumption days. This is usually done by setting five to six "Keto days" (5% carb intake) and one to two "carb loading" days where the carb intake can surge to 60–70%.

The cyclical diet is an advanced type of Keto diet and is only recommended for much more serious athletes such as bodybuilders and other professionals who need a much higher volume and intensity in their workouts or exercises to achieve their optimal performance in their craft. This can also be used by athletes with upcoming competitions who want to boost their training and performance by temporarily upping their carb intake.

To detail this out, during the 5-6 Keto days, the body is forced to burn fats, thus providing a leaner body composition. As for the remaining 1-2 high-carb days, the energy storage of the body is replenished, which can then help in one's training/performance.

Furthermore, this type of Keto diet is also helpful for people who find a hard time sticking with a very strict Keto diet or those who want to take some kind of a "break" in the other types — although this is not to be confused with carelessly carb-binging and entirely jeopardizing one's previous efforts.

On the other hand, the cyclical diet is not suitable for people whose aim is to lose weight or to treat health issues. Also, it is not suitable for people who just casually go to the gym, as this diet needs intense calorie burning workouts and activities to use up the excess carbs.

Research

The Keto diet has been shown to produce advantageous metabolic changes for the short term. Along with weight loss, health issues linked with carrying excess amounts of weight have been included as part of the short-term problems. They would be cholesterol, high blood pressure, and insulin resistance.

There is also an increasing interest as well in the use of low-carb diet types to help with type 2 diabetes. A number of theories are there as to why the Keto diet promotes weight loss, though they have not been consistently affirmed in research.

Comparison with Other High-Efficiency Dietary Plans

There is a variety of high-efficiency weight loss schemes out there that can be brought to this book and compared against the likes of the Keto diet. They include the Paleo diet, Atkins diet, and intermittent fasting.

Atkins Diet

When you are looking for low-carb diet types, the first two that you are most likely going to come across would be the Keto diet and the Atkins diet. You may notice a growing number of comparisons between the two since Atkins is the one most similar to the Keto diet. Both of them use the philosophy of low-carb, high-fat structure—and both of them encourage weight loss. They are not the same, though. For one, the Atkins diet is easier on the carb restrictions, as it allows for moderate carb intake at particular points in time. It is hard for most people considering it is quite different from what people would normally eat. Weight loss is also the main goal when it comes to the Atkins diet, while the Keto diet is focused on overall wellness than anything else. The Keto diet also focuses on switching to a constant state of Ketosis, while the Atkins diet does not lead to serious metabolic changes.

The question for which is more appropriate depends on what you would want to achieve. If you want weight loss, then the Atkins diet is the best option for you. Meanwhile, if you want overall health improvement and weight loss, then the Keto diet would be preferred but is more extreme.

The Paleo Diet

Compared to the Keto diet, the Paleo is much easier. The Paleo diet has thus been seen as much more liberal relative to the Keto diet because there is the availability of more options, and you are going to have more fruits and vegetables. The advantage of the Paleo diet is that it does not enforce strict ratios on the meal structure in the manner that the Atkins and the Keto diet do. Instead, it places a focus on the food groups that one needs to focus on such as meats, vegetables, fruits, and healthy sources of fat.

The basis of the Paleo diet is to avoid things like refined grains and other processed foods. It is basically a way of eating that is similar to the way the early people ate—hence its name making a reference to the Paleolithic era.

Intermittent Fasting

Intermittent fasting is comparable to the Keto diet in the sense that it provides similar benefits to others. There are different ways that one can consider intermittent fasting, though it usually concerns shortening eating window so that the body is not pulling energy from the food being taken in. Then, it becomes forced to utilize the fat stores for the purposes of energy creation. A lot of people do not do this by not eating after certain times in the evening then skipping on breakfast during the morning. Intermittent fasting can be used in combination with keto and can be very effective.

Why You Should Go with the Keto Diet

Each one of these methods allows for you to lose weight, but it is possible that it is because you are eliminating the time given to food and most of the favorite unhealthy foods from the menu, which means that you are not eating as much overall.

The thing is that you may end up losing weight because you have placed a lot of restraints. That being said, if you had to choose one, then the Keto diet would be the best choice out of all of the above. It has been considered by many to give better advantages to the health scheme of the practitioners than most other diets. The Keto diet allows for both weight loss and a better state of health that will keep most lifestyle diseases from occuring. It is also technically healthier, considering you are going to have more options.

Potential Disadvantages

Following a diet rich in fat could be challenging for one to maintain. Some of the symptoms of the Keto diet due to extreme carbohydrate restriction could last from days to weeks—and they include hunger, low moods, fatigue, constipation, and brain fog. Even though these uncomfortable feelings may calm down, staying satisfied with the foods available could bring a few issues. Some of the side effects of taking on a long-term Ketogenic diet include the increased risk of osteoporosis and increased blood levels of uric acid. The potential nutrient deficiencies could come about if a variety of the recommended foods on the Ketogenic diet are not included. It is important for one not to solely focus on the consumption of high-fat foods but to include a variety of the allowed vegetables, meats, fishes, and nuts — this is to ensure the adequate intakes of fiber, minerals, and nutrients found in foods like whole grains. Considering the whole food groups are not included, assistance from a dietician that is verified would be advisable when it comes to the creation of a Ketogenic diet that would minimize the nutrient deficiencies.

As such, though the Ketogenic diet is safe for people who are healthy there are things you would need to deal with. This is usually referred to as the Keto flu and is over within days. In order to minimize the Keto flu, you may try a regular low-carb type diet for the first few weeks in order to teach your body to acclimatize itself to burn fat instead of sugar before eliminating carbs from the diet. A Keto diet would also alter the mineral and water balance of the body — thus, adding salt to the meals or mineral supplements may help with things. For minerals, you can try taking 3000–4000 mg of Sodium, 1000 mg of Potassium, and 300 mg of Magnesium each day to counter the side effects. In the beginning, it would be important to eat until you are full and avoid restricting the calories too much. Usually, the Keto diet would cause some weight loss without internal calorie restrictions.

Myths Concerning the Keto Diet

Here, the book uncovers a number of popular Keto diet myths and sets the record straight to help you decide whether the Keto diet is the right choice for you.

Keto Diet is high in protein.

In order to stay within the state of Ketosis, the ones that are on a Keto diet have to reduce their protein intake. Apparently, when proteins get to a high enough level, the breakdown of the amino acids within the protein may lead to an increase in ketones (substance used for the Ketosis process). That may be well and good to the average dieter — but when it comes to the Keto dieter already with high levels of ketones because of low-carb consumption, it may lead to complications. When the intake of proteins becomes too high, they then become converted to glucose, which then leads to a spike in the blood sugar levels and counters Ketosis.

As such, when you are on a Keto diet, it is important to answer the question: "What is the right amount of protein?" 6 to 8 percent of the daily calories have to come from protein so that one remains in Ketosis and eliminates the risk of complications. For the average woman, that would entail eating about 30 to 40 grams of protein every day. This is equal to two eggs and a 3-ounce chicken breast every day.

Any type of fat is admissible.

The Keto diet may seem like a fat-free for all—but that is not the case, especially if you are thinking of filling up with trans-fats. The replacement of saturated fat such as ham, sausages, and bacon with the unsaturated fats like walnuts and fish is much more effective in reducing the risk of cardiovascular disease rather than reducing the fat consumption overall.

The brain is not able to function properly without carbs.

That time before meals when you are feeling dizzy and irritable is when your blood sugar levels start to reduce completely. At this time, the brain needs glucose as an energy source. At the start of the Keto diet, you may expect for the brain to do a lot of this, which means you will not be pleasant to be around. While research shows that the brain requires about 100 grams of glucose every day in order to function well, the Keto diets allow for an intake of 50 grams of glucose. In the process of becoming adapted with the Keto diet, you are going to go through the same symptoms as you would when you are moody before a meal. Once the body becomes adapted to the Keto diet, the brain will be able to convert ketones to fuel—though some claim that this may take a few months in order to happen.

It is a long-term solution.

For the ones that love fatty foods and are not exceptionally worried about tallying calories and would have the capacity to surrender to carbs easily, the Keto diet would be anything but difficult to keep up over the long haul. The fundamental reason is the more extended that you pursue the Keto diet, the more prominent the danger of muscle loss. Besides contributing to the loss in quality and muscle tone, the reductions in fit muscle mass additionally mean decreases in metabolic rates, which implies that you will consume a less measure of calories — in contrast to when you started to keep off the weight. In spite of the fact that the diet might be profitable for dropping weight quickly, it would be best utilized for just fourteen days on end — for instance, when you are not going hard at the exercise center. In this manner, before expanding the exercise administration, you have to build the measure of carbs and proteins inside your diet.

Chapter 2

GETTING STARTED

For the most obvious reasons, the Keto diet is appealing because it helps people not to stress over their health or bodies and allows them to focus on other things and have the energy to be more effective. There is also the fact that it cures a multitude of health conditions and keeps other significant ones at bay.

Common Mistakes People Make in Keto Diet

In many instances, the Keto diet is approached by people in the wrong manner, which is quite natural for any regiment that is being considered as a cure-all for anything out there. While mistakes are not a big deal, when you are doing Keto, they can have significant effects on your physical or mental state. When beginning the Keto diet, you expect to see results because success is all you see in others that have tried the same thing. When it does not happen the same way, it can be very frustrating for you and lead to a backtracking to carbs. This would be mentally damaging to your diet discipline or perspective. The following are some common perspective and approach mistakes that people make when they engage the Keto diet.

Using the Keto Diet as a Quick Fix

Some people might try and use the diet as a quick fix for their body issues much to their detriment. The diet is not a quick fix but a lifestyle choice that you need to stick by for it to be effective and so you can see a long-term change. You might see some changes happening rather fast but this is not an indication that you can backslide to your original carb filled diet and expect the changes to last. It is very easy to go back to your old ways but that will be a zero-sum game and nothing will be gained in the process.

Being Afraid of Fats

This is a misconception that has been carried over for years by the media and people saying that fat is bad for the body. With this diet, the majority of your consumption is fat which sounds like an oxymoron.

Of course, there are particular fats which are processed which are harmful to the body and these are off limits. Some people might see through that once they have taken into calculation their macros, the amount of fat they have to consume is a lot. On the Keto diet, you have to consume a lot of fat for the body to reach the goals as intended.

Eating Too Much Protein

To some, this seems like the natural thing to do considering you are eliminating carbs from the diet. however, if you have gotten this far in the book then you already know why eating a lot of protein is a bad idea considering they get turned to glucose when carbs are not there and the protein is in plenty. The body only needs a certain amount of protein to function and anything more would be turned into glycogen.

Not Taking Enough Water

When you are on the Keto diet, you lose a lot of fluids through increased urination, this is something that often gets forgotten. It is therefore very easy to get yourself dehydrated or get heart issues because of the loss of electrolytes which would be available if there were enough fluids in the system.

When you are not staying hydrated as well, the body is going to store as much fat as possible as opposed to burning it, so you will need plenty of water to keep the process of Ketosis going.

Not Getting the Right Amount of Sleep

During the Keto diet, when the body starts to use fat as the main source of energy, it is possible to lose some sleep. The advisable thing would be to try to get the right amount of sleep. Not doing this will prevent the body from functioning, as it should especially when it is changing to accommodating the Ketosis.

Looking at the Scale

It is a fact that this diet is geared for you to lose a significant amount of body fat leading to shedding the weight. Though, the fact is that this is a process which is going to take some time and so checking your weight several times during the day or even on a daily basis is going to be frustrating. It is not going to be easy to maintain discipline if you keep doing this. You have to trust the process and that things are going the right way when you stay away from the carbs and hit the macros every day. The weight is eventually going to come off in a steady way. The best thing to do would be to check the weight only once every week to see the progress made.

Key Steps in Getting Started with Keto

The biggest change that comes with the Keto diet, of course, would be the almost complete removal when it comes to carbs from the daily routine. That would usually mean too much change for the majority of people. There are so many mainstream foods out there that would be considered taboo by the Keto diet on account of being composed of the wrong stuff, i.e., carbs. For example, if a big component of your meal consisted of pasta, rice, or bread—you would have to give these up. Now, you are starting to get the picture of how far the diet goes and how intense things can get. So, the first thing that you would do naturally is to find out what you can and cannot eat and then arrange these in a meal format, which would be best for you in the long run.

You will not eat...

- Sugar: honey, maple syrup, and anything processed or which uses sweeteners
- Grain: wheat, corn, cereal, and rice
- Fruit: bananas, apples, and oranges
- Yams and potatoes, which are rich in starch

You can eat...

- Low-carb type of vegetables: leafy greens, broccoli, and others
- Nuts and seeds, walnuts, and sunflower seeds.
- Avocados and other berries, such as raspberries and blackberries
- Sweeteners like monk fruit and stevia
- Fats like saturated fats, coconut oil, and salad dressing

You are most likely going to be able to keep the net carbs and the total level of cholesterol at a low level so that you are able to experience the benefits of low-carb dieting and Ketosis. At any time, if you are uncertain concerning whether a particular food item is Keto-friendly or not, then you can just calculate the net carbs in order to see if it is going to be able to fit within the net carb and total carb limit for the day.

Calculating the Level of Carbs

Restriction of the carb consumption is what is emphasized in the Keto diet because this is how you stay in Ketosis. The first step when it comes to keeping the carbs low would be learning the means of calculating them yourself.

Hence, to get to the net carb structure of any food item, you are going to have to subtract the number of grams of dietary fiber from the number of grams that are represented under total carbohydrates. In equation form, it is going to be:

Total carbs – fiber = net carbs

For that food label, you can calculate the net carbs with an equation, which is 9 grams of the total carbs – 4 grams of the dietary fiber to come up with 5 grams of net carbs every serving. This number is representative of the carbs that are there for every serving. Using this information, you can now assess if a beverage or a food is not friendly when it comes to the Keto diet. If you require assistance with regards to tracking the net carbs throughout the day, then try utilizing a macro app or a chronometer.

Make the Environment Open to the Keto Diet

The level of willpower could be significant at the start, and you may feel like you will have the ability to sail through the new diet plan—however, you have to acknowledge the fact that you are also very human. If the food environment is filled with carb-rich food, which can be found almost everywhere, then even your sheer willpower is not going to stop you from cheating on your diet. In order to make sure that you stick to the Keto plan you set for yourself, you need to supplement willpower with a few helping hands such as making the environment open to Keto. That means taking a break on social outings with people not on the diet and removing food items that are both carb-rich and addictive. Delete all contacts to fast food deliveries, and stock the kitchen with low-carb alternatives if you need to eat snacks. You should also plan meals ahead of time so that you are never left wondering what you want to eat at a particular part of the day.

Prepare for the Keto Flu

This has been mentioned before and is one of the big hurdles that come during the initial stages. If you prepare for it, then it is not going to hit you as hard as it would have if you had just been waiting for it to happen.

The fortunate thing is that a lot of the symptoms are a result of mild dehydration, and they can be remedied with ease through drinking a lot of water or supplementing with the use of potassium, magnesium, and sodium tablets.

Be Mindful of the Amounts of Food That You Are Eating

The intake of calories is that variable that makes the most significant effect with regards to whether you gain or lose weight. For a number of people, restricting on the carbs would be the sufficient thing so that they can lose fat in a consistent manner and spare the loss of muscles. The question remains, though: "What would be the next thing to do when you hit a plateau and when you do not lose that much more weight?" The thing to do would be to go into your calculator and track the levels of calories. In doing this, you will ascertain how much you are eating and how much you need to achieve the goals of body composition. For as long as you are losing weight at a steady rate of 1 or 2 pounds every week, then there is no need to change what you are doing. You will have to assess the levels of progress after every three to five weeks in order to see your overall improvement.

Keto Diet Do's and Don'ts

If you are a rookie in the wonders of the Ketogenic diet, you will soon find out that it is very easy to make mistakes that could keep you from your ultimate goal (whatever it may be) with this diet. While Keto can be used for many purposes including weight loss and fitness, it is just as tricky as any other diet — possibly even trickier, as it calls for maximum fat food intake. Therefore, before you can explore the wonderful world of Keto, take note of the following dos and don'ts — they make a whole lot of difference.

The Do's

1. **Indulge in whole foods.**

One of the best things about Keto is that you will be spoilt for choice in terms of meals because it calls for eating whole foods. Even though the main focus of Keto is fat and protein intake, you will also need a healthy balance of vegetables and fruits to keep things running smoothly in your body. Whole foods basically mean you should eat non-starchy vegetables, nuts, seeds, fresh meat that has been fed grass and is organic, and free of drugs and antibiotics. Because the Keto trend is catching on, you can find packaged meals and Keto restaurants for those days that you cannot cook. These meals are made from whole foods which mean you will be sticking to your diet even if you are too tired to cook.

2. **Hydrate.**

One of the most important things that you should do on a Keto diet is to keep your body well hydrated. Keto draws stored water from cells and causes the kidneys to release more water. As such your usual intake of water will not cut it. While a good amount of water is found in vegetables, you will need additional water especially if you are planning to exercise too. Also, if you drink tea or coffee regular, you should pay close attention to how much water you drink because the caffeine in both is a natural diuretic.

3. Restore electrolytes.

When you start your Keto diet, you will literally be flushing electrolytes down the drain. Because your bathroom habits will have drastically changed in that you will be urinating more often, you will be losing a lot of electrolytes through your urine. The effects of this if not rectified can be dizziness, muscle spasms, headaches, and other inconvenient symptoms. The best way to avoid or stop these symptoms is by replenishing your electrolytes. You can start by adding two teaspoons of natural and high-quality salt to your diet, preferably when cooking. If this is not for you then you can turn to things such as avocados, coconuts, and bone broth to keep your electrolyte levels at the right amount.

4. Check your gut.

The Keto diet is like any other diet you attempt — it is different from your daily routine, and so, you will find yourself experiencing difficulties during the transition. That being said, you should always get your gut checked before, during, and while on the diet. Before you begin your diet, ensure that your doctor clears you for it — people who have experienced difficulties when making the transition often suffer from a type of severe gut complication.

The main cause of this complication is a dietary change that causes you to take more protein or food additives — this is very common with the Keto diet. Other causes include drinking more than two alcoholic beverages per day, accidental consumption of chemicals such as pesticides on vegetables, high levels of stress or anxiety, poor dental hygiene that allows bacteria to grow out of balance inside your mouth, using new medications such as antibiotics that have an effect on the "flora" in your gut, and unprotected sex that exposes you to harmful bacteria.

Symptoms of this complication include an upset stomach, nausea, bad breath, difficulty urinating, severe constipation, bloating, chest pain, fatigue, diarrhea, vaginal and rectal itching, anxiety, a rash or redness on the skin, depression, anxiety, and having trouble thinking and concentrating.

5. **Increase fat intake.**

The Keto diet calls for an increase in the fat you ingest—that way, you will be able to produce ketones. There are five main ways to casually introduce more fat into your diet without overwhelming your gut. First, you can make every hot beverage into a delicious and creamy one. Take your favorite hot beverage—whether tea, coffee, green tea, or hot chocolate—then mix it with your choice of fats, making it as creamy or as foamy as you wish. Fats you can use for this include MCT oil or powder, coconut oil, coconut cream, ghee, butter, and cocoa butter—thus giving you a little chocolate flavor.

The next way you can introduce fats to your diet is through vegetables. Vegetables are an important part of a healthy diet, and while most Keto diet beginners are more concerned with reducing carbohydrates than eating veggies, they are significant to the diet. There is plenty of low-carb, high-fiber vegetables to enjoy while on a Ketogenic diet. Choose a low-carb vegetable such as zucchini, celery, leafy greens, celery, asparagus, cabbage, and broccoli among others. You can also use oil over salads including coconut oil, macadamia nut oil, ghee, butter, and extra virgin olive oil. You should also use high-fat dressings, preferably the type that you make yourself. All you need is an oil base such as extra virgin avocado oil and flavors; some add-ins such as lemon, chili, chives; and finally an additional oil base such as cashews and hemp seeds.

The third way you can introduce fat in Keto is by creating fat bombs. A fat bomb is like any other food bomb; it holds a lovely surprise on the inside. Fat bombs are the best Keto treat because they not only increase your fat intake but also help with the transition into the lifestyle. There are many recipes for fat bombs online, but they all follow the same general ingredients and guidelines. When choosing an ingredient, ensure that it does not contain any added sugars. It is always best to experiment with the best flavors for you—never settle for just one type of bomb. How you keep them depends on the consistency; they can be rolled into balls, or they can be put in silicone sleeve tubes.

The fourth way to introduce fat into your diet is by choosing fatty cuts. Usually, when people pick a meat that they want to consume, they pick the leanest and least fatty cuts. If you are undergoing a Keto diet, the fatty cuts need to become your bread and butter—you can also choose the fatty versions of what you are used to. For example, if you love to eat fishes, you should go for salmon, herring, sardines, and eels. If you are going to have red meat, choose from bison, lamb, and beef. For poultry, enjoy chicken, turkey, and duck—always ensure that the skin remains on for consumption.

The fifth way is through snacking on fatty snacks. Regular diets encourage you to snack on healthy vegetable snacks such as carrots. However, this is not the case with a Keto diet—the diet encourages you to snack on high-fat foods such as macadamias, boiled eggs, avocado, pecans, and dairy products. This introduces more fat into your diet without overwhelming your digestive tract.

6. Try different approaches.

There are many rules in the Keto diet, and you may find yourself struggling to maintain the rules while still finding a system that works for you. At the end of the day, the diet should cause more good than harm. That being said, it is imperative that you try out different methods and systems within the diet until you find what works best for you. This is because what works for one person may not necessarily work for the other — and while you think you are doing what someone else did because it worked, you could be missing out on an opportunity to maximize your results with the diet. Also, you should take a close look at your health or any abnormal changes, then consult a nutritionist to make the necessary changes so as to not harm you. More importantly, you can always get help and information from trained professionals, tutorials, and self-help books.

The Don'ts

1. Say no to processed food.

Your main aim, while you are on this diet, is to avoid carbohydrates as much as possible. Carbohydrates are primarily present in processed foods which can be a little difficult to avoid completely. Many processed foods are also filled with chemicals and preservatives that are toxic to your diet and can slow down the process of reaching Ketosis. Labels such as 'low-carb', and 'sugar-free', should be avoided regularly as well as unhealthy fats in the form of corn oil, canola oil, vegetable oil, and hydrogenated oil.

2. Avoid overeating.

One of the best things about the Keto diet is that the meals are quite satisfying and filling. What's more is that even when you feel full, you will have consumed fewer calories as compared to eating a meal rich in carbohydrates. During the first few days, you will find yourself serving proportions as you would with a carb-filled meal in order to feel full. However, if you feel full, you should not feel obligated to finish the meals as you would be taking in more calories than you need which would be stored as fat. Therefore, if you are satisfied, do not overeat.

3. Avoid too much dairy.

On paper, there is nothing wrong with dairy or nuts because they are healthy, and a source of water and fiber. However, they are extremely calorie-dense meaning that they have a high number of calories per 100 grams. It is quite easy to find yourself over-indulging in these two and may trigger you into over-eating. Therefore, if you feel that they may cause you to overeat, take keen note of how much you eat and reduce consumption to once in a while or at least once every two weeks.

4. Do not guess.

While you may think you understand what each food is composed of, you may not fully grasp what it actually means. Most people guess what food is considered 'organic' or 'good fat' then end up eating something that is completely off their diet plan. If you are unsure about a particular food, rather than guess; you should look it up and do research on it so you can determine whether you should eat it. If you do not want to make that kind of call, then you can always ask for help from nutritionist's and dieticians so you do not unknowingly cheat on your diet.

5. **Avoid exogenous ketones.**

Because the Keto diet has become so popular, people started making Ketogenic supplements. Exogenous supplements come from a synthetic source, unlike endogenous ketones which are produced by the body when you are on a Keto diet. The most common is Keto salts; they are a powdered supplement made with a Ketone molecule bound to one of several mineral salts such as calcium, sodium, potassium, and magnesium. Another popular form is the Ketone Esters; they are salt-free liquids in one (monoester), two (diester), and three (triester) form. This means that rather than being bound to a mineral like calcium, the Ketone molecule is bound to a

Ketone precursor such as glycerol and Butanediol through an ester bond. Esters are less popular than salts and the ones that exist have some variance.

So why should you not use the supplements if they are available? For starters, a serving of exogenous ketones will just end up setting you back 100 calories. Secondly, they have a really bad taste, so you might aswell eat something alot tastier instead. What is more, the supplements are expensive; a two week supply of the stuff could cost you up to 50 dollars, money which would be better spent on whole foods. Keto salts pose a danger to your body because they are bound to minerals such as sodium; these are dangerous for people who have high blood pressure. This could create problems with the health of the heart and how it functions.

Another issue is that the supplements could cause stomach distress; if your gut is not strong, the supplements can possibly disturb it. An entire serving is enough to give you serious tummy troubles for over a week. Considering ketones are a sign that your body is burning fat, adding Ketone supplements to your diet will not allow you to lose weight if that is your goal.

6. **Do not worship fast food.**

When people hear that the Keto diet calls for high-fat foods, the first thing they think about is fast food. While burgers and fries do have a high concentration of fat, they should not be all you eat; in fact, if you can avoid them you really should. Instant burgers and fries are not your best option because they are laden with preservatives and chemicals that will prevent you from reaching a state of Ketosis.

Chapter 3

HOW THE KETO DIET WORKS

Why do we get fat? It is one of those questions people ask but never really think about, yet it is something that happens in everyday life. In order to understand how Keto affects the body, we must first understand how and why we get fat. Over the past ten years, science has narrowed down the fault of weight gain and loss to a hormone known as Leptin. Leptin is a hormone within the fat cells. Its job is to alert your brain when you are full. It is an important signal, but for many, it is not working—thanks to insulin. Insulin as a significant hormone has higher signal levels than almost any other in the body. The task of this hormone is to convert blood sugar into body fat.

The nourishment we eat is important in furnishing the body with the fuel or vitality utilized for everyday exercises. Despite the fact that they both keep running on some type of engine, bodies are unique in relation to cars. While cars just keep running on gasoline, bodies are intended to utilize three principle fills to function—sugars, protein, and fats. Starches are the essential segment of starch, sugars, and flour, which are regularly present in plants. Proteins mostly come from animals and are represented by meat and fish. A few plants—for example, beans and different vegetables—are likewise great sources of protein. Fats come in two primary varieties: unsaturated fats like corn oil and saturated fats such as a spread that originated from animal parts.

These three fuel types all experience a similar response—they intertwine with the oxygen we inhale to produce vitality to be utilized by the body and waste items—for example, pee and carbon dioxide. This is like when a car burns fuel or when we burn wood and coal for warmth. Despite the fact that each of the three nutrition classes is used in a similar way, starches are utilized first, trailed by fats, and lastly by proteins. Overall, sugars will be utilized inside a couple of hours after they are eaten. So what are the end results for unused sugars? They are stored in the liver as fat reserves.

The most basic job of fats is to store vitality. The body typically stores the fats that we eat. On the off chance that there isn't sufficient supply of sugars, the body will attempt to amend this by separating the fat stored to use as fuel for. However, fats are utilized substantially more gradually than carbs. This is the motivation behind why individuals feel fuller after a greasy feast when contrasted with a low-sugar supper. The other fuel, protein, is utilized to supplant and repair body materials and muscle. Excess protein is processed as fuel for the body or discharged. On the off chance that in any case starches and fat stores are totally exhausted, the body will begin to separate muscle with the end goal to utilize the protein for fuel in an endeavor to spare itself. In an essential Western diet, the extent by weight of how the three powers are utilized is 5 to 15% proteins, 10 to 20% fat, and 65 to 85% starches. Any excesses will be stored in the body as fat or will be discharged. This, as you will see, is totally not quite the same as the Ketogenic diet.

Chapter 4

FATS, CARBS, AND PROTEINS

As noted, protein, carbs, and fats are the three constituents of every Keto-aligned meal — though they are set according to different levels. The protein levels should be higher than the carbs, and the fats should be twice as high as either of them in every meal. The basis of this chapter is to give a chance to consider the types of each group that are admissible, as definitely not all fats nor all proteins would be considered within the Keto diet.

The Importance of Fat When It Comes to the Keto Diet

Dietary fat is the main element in the Keto diet. It is the high intake of fat and low amount of carb consumption, which leads to the success of the diet and the initiation of Ketosis where the brain and the body use ketones for fuel, burning through the fat stores in the body. Having a low intake of carbs allows you to go through the stores of carbs within the body — not to mention the stored carbohydrates — conditions the body to begin turning to fat, which allows for the creation of ketones for energy. Keeping the body within the state of Ketosis has a lot of advantages, which would entail weight loss and a better state of well-being.

Calorie Intake Is Significant.

The ones new to the Keto diet or those who have taken a break from it tend to struggle with consuming the right amount of fat at the beginning. Because one is reducing the carb consumption, you would have to increase the amount of fat eaten in order to replace the calories that you were eating previously from the carbs. If you are not used to eating high levels of healthy fats, then it could be intense at the start. Fat is satiating and this is one of the advantages of the Keto diet considering you may naturally be able to avoid being able to overeat because of the way it is satisfying. That being said it is also crucial for one to eat a sufficient amount of calories while on the Ketogenic diet so that you can avoid thyroid or metabolic issues which are linked with low-calorie intake and do more harm as opposed to good. Though the low-calorie intake may assist during the beginning for the reduction of body fat, it would be problematic over the long term.

How to Increase Fat Intake?

You will have to find out how many grams this comes to by using a calculator in order to ascertain the daily calorie intake. From there, you can place these percentages to ascertain the amount of protein and grams of fat which you would require and then you will get the baseline of how much is required each day. In an example, a person that consumes 2000 calories each day and a fat intake of 70 to 80 percent would be at 144 grams to 177g grams of fat every day. If the calories that are needed are greater, then you may need even more than that.

Sources of Healthy Fats

There are different places where one can get fat when they are doing the Ketogenic diet. The best resources would be the whole foods that carry monounsaturated fats. These include pasture raised eggs, coconut and avocado oil, nuts and seeds, fatty cuts of some meats, butter, fatty fish and cocoa butter. Besides the regular tracking of the number of calories and fat, and carbs that are being consumed every day to make certain that you are eating enough of each, it would be good to proceed with testing and monitoring of the Ketone levels.

Daily Protein Requirements

The official recommended allowance daily for protein intake is usually set at 0.36 grams per pound of your weight each day. The protein needs for the ones that want to optimize their health or are on a low-carb diet like Keto would be different. It is significant to know that the daily protein requirements should not have to be based on the calorie percentage. The protein requirements of an individual are constant regardless of the number of calories that they eat every day considering the protein needed relates to a function of the lean body mass of the individual or on the ideal body weight. Calculation of the protein needs ought to be based according to the maintenance of a good nitrogen balance. Amino acids have nitrogen, and the protein that is consumed becomes metabolized into amino acids for utilization when it comes to building new muscle and other tissues. Excess nitrogen may be excreted through the urine.

When the amount that is excreted happens to be less than the amount of nitrogen in the food that you have eaten, then you can say that you are in a good nitrogen type balance. If you do not take enough protein, then you may get into a negative type of nitrogen balance. That would be that you are using internal protein sources in order to cover the shortage of protein that occurs within the diet. The bottom line when it comes to the negative nitrogen balance scenario is you lose lean body mass which is not the intended purpose.

Some of the proteins allowed during the Keto diet include some of the following though they are to be taken in moderation:

- Fish, especially if it is of the fatty variety such as salmon.
- Grass-fed or non-GMO beef and other meats.
- Dark meat chicken

At times, you have the chance to indulge in bacon diets, low-fat proteins like skinless chicken and shrimp. Proteins which are not included in the list for the Keto diet include meat which has been marinated in sugar sauces, and fish or chicken nuggets.

Good and Bad Foods and Drinks to Consume on Keto

It is not a secret that the changing dietary lifestyle takes a bit of time and planning. The knowledge of the best foods that one can eat when they are on the Keto diet is going to allow for you to be prepared for a smoother type of transition and better results in the long run.

Meat

Unprocessed meat is usually low-carb and Keto friendly though as mentioned before the organic and grass-fed type is the healthiest option of all. You need to remember though that Keto is high-fat and not particularly high protein which means protein would be served in moderate amounts. Excess protein would be converted to glucose and become counterproductive. Note the fact that processed meats including cold cuts, meatballs usually contain carbs added to them. Look at the ingredients if in doubt and aim for something that has a carb percentage of less than 5%.

Eggs

These can be eaten in any way, especially boiled, fried in butter, scrambled or as omelets however you would prefer. You may try and buy organic for the healthiest alternative. The best thing to do in this case would be to have no more than 36 eggs every day. Though, you should feel free to eat fewer of them if you need to.

Natural Fat and High-Fat Sauces

A lot of the calories on the Keto diet need to come from fat. It will be better to get a lot of it from natural sources such as meat, fish, and eggs. Though, you also need to utilize fat when it comes to cooking such as butter or coconut oil. You may also eat delicious high-fat sauces.

Fish and Seafood

These are good especially the fatty type of fish such as salmon. Though, you should avoid adding bread crumbs to them as you would be infusing carbs to the mix. If it is possible to get wild caught fish, then that would be the best option for the Ketogenic diet.

Vegetables That Are Grown Above Ground

Fresh or frozen vegetables are the best option. You can choose vegetables growing above ground particularly the leafy and green ones. You can also consider favorites like cabbage, avocado, broccoli, and zucchini. Vegetables are some of the great and tasty ways of eating good fat when you are on the Keto diet. You can fry them using butter or use a lot of olive oil on your salad and it would be okay. It is weird to think of vegetables as a fat delivery system. They tend to add more flavor, variety, and color to the Keto meal structure. You may find that you end up eating up more vegetables than before when beginning the Keto considering the vegetables would replace the rice, pasta, and potatoes.

Nuts

These can be taken in a state of moderation though you need to be careful when you are using nuts as snacks considering it can be easy for you to eat more than you require to feel satisfied. You should also note that cashews are relatively high on the carb scale so they are not the best option. You are better off opting for macadamia or pecan nuts.

High-Fat Dairy

A high level of fat is good for this particular scenario. Interestingly yogurt and butter are good while high-fat cheese is okay though the yogurt and the cheese would have to be taken in moderation. Heavy amounts of cream are also good for cooking. You need to avoid taking milk as well because as milk sugar adds up to increase the level of carbs that are being taken. Though, it is permissible to use it in a sparing manner such as using it in coffee. You would have to avoid such things as cafe latte and low-fat yogurts which have a number of added sugars.

Coffee

When there is no sugar and a small amount of milk or cream added to eat, then this would be okay. For extra energy, you can try to stir in butter and coconut oil. Though if weight loss stalls then you can cut back on the creams or the fats within your coffee.

Tea

Even if it is green or black, mint or herbal you should feel free to drink tea provided you do not add sugar.

Bone Broth

These tend to be hydrating and satisfying as they have a lot of electrolytes and nutrients. Bone broth is very beneficial as a beverage to sip whilst your on the Keto diet so you can stir it in some extra butter if you need the extra energy.

Grains

These are among the public enemy number ones when it comes to the Keto diet because they are choc-full of carbs. That means any food which derives from grain such as bread and flour is not on the Keto optimal foods list. Some of the foods that you would have to abstain from include pasta, cereal, rice, and bread.

Thoughts on Good vs. Bad Carbs

The usual way of grouping carbs would either be in the form of the good or as the bad variety. This is mostly dependent on whether the carbs themselves have been refined or in the event they are within their natural state. Refining makes them bad, as it reduces the nutritional value of the food, which then leaves you with a source of calories that are not going anywhere. When it comes to bad carbs, the biggest issue when it comes to refining would be the loss of apparent fiber. Fiber is indigestible as a carbohydrate, which is significant for your health needs. It slows the digestion of the carbs themselves and the blood glucose levels that are out of balance. When one eats bad carbs, which do not have a lot of fiber, the blood sugar levels go up and down in a dramatic manner. These fluctuations when it comes to the levels of blood glucose can place you at a risk of type 2 diabetes if it is not checked on. There are some nutritionists who are of the idea that carbs can either be classified as either good or bad considering the levels of their complexity. The complex-nature carbs are the ones that are considered good, while the simple ones are the bad carbs. However, this is where many people do not agree on the same thing. Simple carbs such as fructose exist in fruit, though most of them would not really call a fruit something that can cause harm.

Bad Carbs While on the Keto Diet (Sugars and Starch)

The Keto diet is very different when compared to the standard diet for many people—i.e. it operates on a different system of determining what is good and bad. For example, when on a Keto diet, fat is actually good, while carbs are mostly bad. Protein is good but only to a certain degree. Sugars are typically frowned upon—thus, nectar, honey, table sugar, and brown sugar should all be avoided. The reason is that they raise the blood glucose levels instantly and to a great extent. You should try to only use sweeteners that will not affect your levels of sugar in the blood or contribute to your intake of carbs.

Condiments, Herbs, and Spices

When it comes to topping the meals on the Keto diet, homemade is the recommended path to take. When possible, it would be advisable to make your versions of the particular spices and other condiments to keep at your residence. That being said, life can get hectic, so you may not have the time to experiment with every healthy combination. Some of the options available, though, would include anchovy paste, Capers, clam juice, unsweetened cocoa powder, and fish sauce. You may dress with lemon juice, oil, vinegar, or ranch dressing as an alternative.

A number of traditional seasonings and sauces are not particularly friendly to the Keto diet, as they have added sugars and starch—thus, herbs and spices become the go-to to make the food better. Some of the potential spaces you may use with food include thyme, oregano, basil, cayenne pepper, cumin, chili powder, and cilantro.

Alcohol and the Keto Diet

Having a social life may be somewhat challenging, considering carbs are very mainstream—and it is hard to find a meal plan when you are eating out with friends that are not going to compromise the diet. This is especially the case when you are out for a drink with friends. Cutting out the wine and the beer for starters would be advisable. Stick to hard liquor if you have to drink because they basically have zero calories in most cases.

There are reports that drinking hard liquor may even deepen the level of Ketosis—though, on the other hand, it does slow down the process of weight loss. Ingesting alcohol has an effect on the liver metabolism in which more of the ketones are produced as you drink more. You should note that a number of people experience a heightened level of being drunk on the Keto diet or getting high quicker than usual. That may just have to do with the fact, though, that hard liquor is involved. That may be the desired effect for some, but you need to be careful especially if you have other things to do with the day like driving or operating machinery. There are a lot of people that experience a very harsh hangover while going to the Keto diet, so you need to ensure that you stay hydrated. The advice would be to take a glass of water for every shot or glass of alcohol taken—as impractical as that may seem.

You may opt for wines and beers low on the carbs, which you can try if you are not the type for hard liquor. You may consider Miller 64, Bud Select, or Michelob Ultra in the case of the beers; and unsweetened champagne, dry red wine, or dry white wine for the wines, which are very low on carbs. That being said, if you can avoid taking alcohol while on the Keto diet, then this would be a lot better, as the results will be less complicated.

Chapter 5

HEALTH BENEFITS & POSSIBLE SIDE EFFECTS OF KETO

Health Benefits

The Keto diet is credited as one of the fastest ways of losing weight, though research suggests that a number of other benefits are there with this low-carb and high-fat method. This chapter considers the benefits of using the Keto diet, along with the potential side effects, which can be experienced by individuals.

Low-carb diets kill appetite.

Hunger is a side effect when you are trying different diets because the body is not getting what it's used to most of the time. It is one of the reasons why people get moody, feel miserable and sad, and eventually give up on the diet, as their dependencies on sugar may be very high. One of the good things about eating a low-carb diet is that it is going to quickly lead to an automatic reduction in appetite, especially if you supplement it with a high-fat intake. Research is showing that when you remove carbs from the diet and opt for more fat and protein, you end up consuming a lower number of calories.

Bigger proportions of the fat lost are from the abdominal space.

Not all fat in the body is the same. It is where the fat is stored that determines how it is going to affect your health and the potential for disease. There is subcutaneous fat under the skin and also visceral fat that lies within the abdominal cavity. Visceral fat is the one that is lodged around the organs. Having fat in this location may increase the level of inflammation and resistance for insulin, and it is believed it is one of the major drivers for metabolic dysfunction, which is very common in Western states in the present. Low-carb-oriented diets are quite effective when it comes to the reduction of abdominal fat, for example. Not only do they cause things such as fat loss as compared to the low-fat diets, but a great percentage of the fat burned up is from the abdominal cavity. Over the course of time, that would lead to a much-reduced risk of type 2 diabetes and heart disease.

Low Blood Sugar

Obviously, when you wean yourself from sugars, the blood sugar is going to drop. Lowering the insulin levels as a result of the running off of ketones allows you to control and lower the level of blood sugar. The chance to utilize ketones as the fuel source for the body is to mean that the diabetic or the type-2 diabetic does not have to worry concerning excess blood sugar.

There was a study done in 1976 that illustrated the way type 2 diabetic patients on the Ketogenic diet did not need insulin, and they, as a result, lost a lot of body weight. The findings were then backed by a study in 2012 that had diabetic patients that were obese go along with a Ketogenic diet for a period of 12 months.

Weight Loss

High-fat and low-carb diets have been used for several hundreds of years by doctors when working with patients that are obese. One of the main reasons why the Keto diet has become so popular is that it is associated with notable weight loss. It is an easily recognizable effect on the body for obvious reasons. Because the Ketogenic diet calls for higher intake of fats, you will feel fuller, which results in lower levels of cravings, more self-control in what you eat, a lower calorie intake, and surprisingly, a greater need to do physical activities. These all eventually lead to weight loss. Because you have stopped or reduced the number of carbohydrates you eat every day, there is less glucose to be burned for fuel and even less to be stored as fat. This causes the body to use the fats in the food you eat or the ones that are already stored in your body to burn and use as fuel. As a result, your fat deposits will get smaller and smaller until they are fully depleted, and the body starts to rely on the fats you will eat. Ketosis is a built-in mechanism because if you begin to starve, the body will immediately start to use up fats stored for fuel. It is the reason why people who are starving lose weight rapidly. If the cycle continues without a regular intake of fats, the body will begin to use the proteins in muscle as fuel. This is why if you are looking to build on muscle on a Ketogenic diet, you should include high amounts of fats as well as proteins to prevent the body from digging into your body-building proteins.

A lot of people successfully use the Keto diets at the present in their quest for decreased levels of body fat for the same reasons. Through consumption of a high-fat and low-carb diet, you get to retrain the systems to utilize fat as the energy source — and that makes the body start to burn up its reserves of fat to create energy in the process of Ketosis. If you have a lot of fat around your organs or in your skin and abdominal area, then it can be a great way to lose weight symmetrically.

Brain Function

Other than the loss of fat, one of the reasons why a number of people continue to rave concerning the Keto diets is because of improved levels of brain functions and improved learning. Science backs these claims as a study done on rats found the Keto diet led to a cognitive improvement in rats which were elderly. A study done on people came to the conclusion that Keto diets even when used during the short term allowed for the improvement of memory in elderly people especially. The Keto diet was also shown to increase things like the ATP concentrations. Anyone that has done the Keto diet successfully will tell you there are significant cognitive benefits to be had by having a state of Ketosis.

The sugar found in your blood known simply as glucose is the main fuel used by the brain. It powers up the brain to be able to control the whole body including major organs such as the heart, respiratory organs, and the digestive system. Without said fuel, the brain would shut down and would be followed suit by the other major and minor organs. In the event where glucose levels have seemingly dropped either on purpose or accidentally, the brain will switch to backup power because surprisingly, the brain loves fat. In a Ketogenic diet, your liver produces ketones, these ketones are essential for proper brain function where glucose is in short supply. Reports have shown that people on a Keto diet have shown remarkable improvement in verbal skills and their memories seem sharper. It is why many nutritionists say that fat is a well-known brain food especially the ones present in monosaturated fats such as nuts, seeds, and olive oil. When carbohydrates are eliminated, ketones provide up to 70% of the energy used by the brain. It is important to note however that there are some parts of the brain that will still need glucose to function properly. On an extremely low-carb diet, more glucose can be made through a process called gluconeogenesis which roughly translates to 'making new glucose'. In this process, the liver creates the glucose for the brain to use through breaking down amino acids.

Endurance Performance

If you are an endurance type of athlete and you have not considered the benefits of Ketosis and endurance performance them, you are missing out on what may be a big edge in your game. The research done on endurance sports and Ketosis paints a very optimal picture. The results claim that the ones on a Keto diet had more mitochondria as compared to the control group which means they experienced a lower level of oxidative stress and a lower lactate load so athletes could function off fat for a higher intensity as compared to those non-fat adapted people. Clearly, this would be advisable for those who are running marathons or trying out for the military as the body will be at a lower level of adaptive stress and allow you a higher threshold of pain to complete the objectives as compared to others.

Stable Levels of Energy

When you eat a meal rich in carbohydrates, the glucose will be burned to produce energy. In order to achieve this, the body will produce insulin from the pancreas to move the glucose from your bloodstream and into the cells. Therefore, as the levels of glucose rise after mashed potatoes, insulin starts being released to ensure that your heart has the energy to pump blood. This process essentially helps to lower your blood sugar levels and once your body has had enough energy, it sends a signal to the liver and other muscle tissues to store the glucose for later. The insulin sends another signal to the liver to inform it that your glucose stores are full. If you have insulin sensitivity, then your body will struggle to absorb the energy and will probably need more insulin to handle the task. Often, you will be left with excess glucose in your bloodstream which gives you an immediate surge in energy followed by a huge drop in the opposite direction popularly known as 'crashing'. This leaves you feeling sluggish and craving more energy in the form of sugar and carbohydrates.

Any individual that has recently switched from the standard western carb filled diet to the Keto diet is going to soon notice the way their energy levels are stable during the course of the day without spikes or sudden lows. There will not be any mid-afternoon slumps or cravings for sugar or caffeine as well. The fat is readily available within your body and from the food that you consume. It also does not come with particular cravings like the way sugar holds the brain ransom in order for the body to generate fuel. Once a person is fat adapted and in a state of Ketosis, they will see that they can easily go for hours or days without having food and they will not suffer from drastic energy level swings. If an individual is looking for a non-caffeine or non-sugar type of kick while they are in a state of Ketosis, then Ketone salts which act as supplements would be the best answer.

In a Ketogenic diet, the body becomes very efficient at burning excess fats for energy. Because ketones do not function in the same way as glucose, there will be no excess insulin produced, and so your body will not have any leftover glucose. The ketones being used for energy instead give you a steady and stable energy surge with no ups or down. Your energy will be consistent and on a controlled level.

Migraine Treatment

A number of people that suffer from severe headaches and migraines have claimed good results when they switch from what would be a conventional high-carb diet to the Keto option. It is also not just the anecdotal evidence which is illustrating the connection between Ketosis and the treatment of migraines. A study that was published within the Journal of Headache pain was of the opinion that Keto diets alleviate headaches and migraine for the short term.

Low-carb diets are therapeutic for brain disorders.

It is claimed that glucose is needed for the brain and that is actually a fact. Some parts of the brain are only able to burn glucose to operate. Though, an even bigger portion of the brain is able to burn ketones that are created during starvation or when the levels of carbs are low. That is the concept behind the Keto diet and it has, for example, been used to treat those children who are suffering from epilepsy. A lot of the time this diet can cure children that are suffering from epilepsy. Studies have illustrated that over half of the groups in experiments entailing Keto diets had a reduction in seizures which is to say that it verily improves the brain functioning and processes. As a result, the Ketogenic diet is being investigated for its effects on other brain disorders such as Parkinson's and Alzheimer's.

Better Sleep Patterns

Many who are on the Keto diet have reported that they sleep much better. On the other hand, at the time of the adjustment period which is the first three to five days after beginning the Keto diet, there may be some insomnia or difficulty staying asleep. This is going to end once the body adjusts to the state of Ketosis and burning of the stored fat. Then you are going to find that you have the ability to sleep better and for a longer periods of time. You will also probably feel more relaxed and rested by the time that you get up in the morning.

Reduction of Inflammation Issues/Marks

Physicians are able to measure the levels of inflammation within the body with the use of blood tests for high sensitivity C reactive proteins and the counts of white blood cells in the body. Apparently, patients are more likely to experience a reduction in the reactive proteins and a reduction in the white blood cell count. Inflammation is related to a number of health conditions such as autoimmune conditions, arthritis, and diabetes and so it is possible to reduce the rate of inflammations through the means of nutritional Ketosis which could then improve a number of conditions in the process.

Healthier Liver

The accumulation of fat within the liver is related to type 2 diabetes or pre-diabetes. In serious cases, the fatty liver disease may lead to damage to the liver. Doctors test for the condition by measuring the levels of the enzymes in the liver via a number of blood tests. These enzymes tend to reduce after some time in clinical patients and that means a less risk of developing fatty liver disease. If you have been informed that you have the risk of getting the fatty liver disease, then you might want to give the diet plan a go.

Mood Stabilization for Autism and Bipolar Disorders

It would seem the Keto stabilizes brain operations in more ways than one by altering the brain chemistry to the advantage of the patient. If you search research on Ketosis and autism, there will be hundreds of results of statements and articles where people have provided testimony on the way it has improved autism while on the Keto diet. One particular study focused on 30 children doing the Keto diet. Those children on the lower end of the spectrum with mild autism are the ones that experienced the most improvement according to the study. The rest of the patients still displayed some improvement though it was mild to moderate in these cases. There are also a number of reports which claim the Keto diet aids with such things like mood stabilization in those people that are suffering from bipolar disorders.

It Is Easier to Fast.

When on the Keto diet, you give up on a lot of those foods which you craved and practices such as binge eating because it reduces the capacity for overeating. Thus one of the best ways to get into a state of Ketosis would be through fasting. Though anyone that is indulging on a high-carb diet would be very afraid if they had to go through 12 hours or longer without. Unfortunately, that is what carbs do as they make the brain demand for food at a few hours at a time even when it is unnecessary. Yet, once you become fat adapted and you are in a state of nutritional Ketosis, then fasting becomes very easy. You can go even 16 hours without needing to eat anything and that is not necessarily sitting in one place. You can do a variety of activities without the body demanding a pound of flesh to go on.

Irritable Bowel Syndrome

A number of people that suffer from irritable bowel syndrome which entails bloating, stomach discomfort and chronic diarrhea consume foods which they are allergic or sensitive toward. The reduction of carbs from their diet places lesser stress on their digestive systems.

Increasing the fat intake may lead to increased diarrhea in the beginning though but the long-term effects of the diet include stabilization and easing of the symptoms.

Anti-Aging

The lowering of the oxidative stress in the body is one of the better ways that one can increase their lifespan apparently. It would seem that through lowering the levels of insulin, the oxidative stress would then be decreased. The Keto diet reduces the levels of insulin and allows one to form ketones so they could be used as fuel. A number of experts are also turning to the Keto diets so as to slow the process of aging. This is upcoming within the scientific field and should prove beneficial for those who want to slow down their aging process without having to spend thousands of dollars on cosmetic surgery and recovery.

Cancer

The process of Ketosis has been proven to be a deterrent to cancer and is a treatment option which is gradually increasing in popularity. The reason is a number of cancer patients are reporting large benefits when they follow the Keto diet. The reason is cancer cells tend to survive only on glucose cells as their source of fuel. Through depriving the cancer cell of glucose when doing the Keto diet, then you may be able to starve cancer thus resulting in its death. Science is also gradually catching up and relating the Keto diets as a form of cancer therapy.

A feasibility research study was done on 10 cancer patients in 2012. The patients went with the Keto diet for a period of 28 days after they exhausted every treatment option for their condition. The findings were there was 1 partial remission of cancer. 5 of the patients stabilized and 4 of them continued progressing. It is crucial to note that these people had tried every other form of cancer treatment. About 60 percent of these individuals then improved or stalled their rates of cancer through following the Keto diet.

Acne

There is a lot of evidence emerging that Ketosis would assist in clearing acne. Foods that have a high glycemic index apparently stimulate breaks of acne and as the Ketogenic diet does without rich foods, it would make sense that it would have a positive effect on acne. There is research which has illustrated a positive relation between Ketosis and acne reduction though it is not yet conclusive evidence to show that Ketosis reduces the severity and progression of acne and randomized clinical trials in order to resolve the problem.

Potential Side Effects of the Keto Diet

Many people are quickly jumping on Keto because of the benefits and because it surprisingly encourages the ingestion of fats over carbohydrates. However, there are a number of effects that Keto makes on the body—some are easily recognizable and obvious, while others will require somewhat a trained eye. If you are new to the diet, you are bound to notice many changes to your body—the majority are considered strange but beneficial. A small percentage of these effects may not necessarily work in your favor, but they are normal to experience and are often manageable. It is important to note that if you notice anything out of the ordinary, you should consult a doctor immediately.

The Keto diet requires one to adhere to what would otherwise be stressful regiments for low-carb and high-fat meals. There are a lot of advantages to this as has been covered, but every good thing comes with its side effects, especially for such an extreme dietary plan.

Inflammation

Inflammation is an important step in the body trying to heal itself and stay protected from any form of illness and injury or damage. However, it is popularly known that too much inflammation can cause serious problems to the body. One of the effects of a Ketogenic diet is that its been proven to reduce inflammation. Being in a state of Ketosis means that the body utilizes fat instead of glucose — and in order to understand this, it is important to note that glucose raises inflammation markers and makes free radicals, which are the molecules that can inflame blood vessel linings and stimulate the immune response of the body. In a Ketogenic diet, the production of insulin is halted because of the low glucose intake, which is said to block out certain types of inflammations.

Bad Breath

This is one of the most common effects of a Keto diet on the body and one that does not particularly work in your favor. If you have been on a Keto diet before, you may have noticed that after you have achieved Ketosis, your breath will immediately start to smell; if you have never been on this diet, then expect bad breath when you start to get into it. There are two possible causes of bad breath when on a Keto diet. The first is as a result of Ketone release. With a very low-carb diet, the body is unable to utilize glucose as a fuel. As a result, the body will produce ketones, which, when produced in large quantities, will prompt the body to discharge the excess through urine—and more commonly through exhalation. Usually, ketones have a very distinct smell and will make the person's breath smell fruity and even quite sweet. However, in large quantities, the smell is very different—it ends up smelling like you drank several bottles of nail polish remover.

Keto Rash

A Keto rash is a very rare inflammatory condition on the skin that is characterized by a red and itchy rash around the trunk and neck areas. It is a type of dermatitis that can occur in anyone who is on the diet but is quite common in Asian women—specifically, as research has shown young Japanese women to fall victim of it. The symptoms include an itchy red rash primarily on the upper back, chest, and abdomen; red spots that appear as a web-like pattern; and finally, a dark brown pattern on the skin after the spots have disappeared.

A lot of the suspected causes for the Keto rash are concerning the creation of ketones like being on the standard Ketogenic diet, losing weight, fasting, or being pregnant, as the latter usually go in and out of Ketosis when they are sleeping. On the other hand, the Keto rash problem could be perceived in the wrong way. It is known that on the Keto diet, the acetone can be excreted through the skin in the form of sweat. If you are an active individual, then it could be possible that the Ketone body excretion is the reason behind the rash.

Urine

One of the major effects of a Ketogenic diet on your body will be most present in your urine. Most people do not take any interest in looking at or examining their urine; it is a bodily waste that is considered disgusting to look at (even when it is yours).

As the body continues to burn through the stored glucose within the liver and the muscles within the initial days of the Keto diet, you will be releasing lots of water through urination. The kidneys will also begin to excrete excess amounts of sodium as the levels of the circulating insulin go down. As such, you may notice that you need to urinate more often during the day. This side effect takes care of itself, though.

The Keto Flu

The Keto flu is one of those effects of the Keto diet on your body that will not work in your favor. The body is accustomed to burning glucose for fuel—when that supply of glucose becomes scarce, the body will burn fat instead. The body's natural reaction to the switching from glucose to fat burning is what is known as the Keto flu.

The body's response to entering the state of Ketosis would be to mimic symptoms of the flu such as diarrhea, nausea, stomach pains, dizziness, confusion, and heart palpitations, among others. In an in-depth analysis, the Keto flu is as a result of three main things; becoming 'Keto-adapted', electrolyte loss and dehydration, and withdrawal from carbohydrates and sugary foods.

The Basic western diet consists of a lot of processed foods that are high in sugars and have a lot of added salts. When you switch to a Keto diet, a lot of that salt is no longer ingested, and so, your sodium intake is reduced dramatically. Because sodium makes the body retain water, less sodium intake means that you will urinate more often. With the excess water being released from your cells and kidneys, electrolytes are also being flushed out. This leads to an electrolyte imbalance and, of course, dehydration. The body will start to depict flu-like symptoms until the levels of electrolytes become balanced again.

Recent research has shown that sugar has the same effect on the brain as cocaine to some extent. When you ingest sugar, you are likely to experience the effects of dopamine, the 'feel good' hormone. The effect of cutting back on sugar in your diet is similar to that of a cocaine addict suddenly stopping. With this, the body will experience withdrawal effects similar to that of the flu—including mood swings, craving sugar, and irritability.

Constipation

This is an adverse effect of the Keto diet on your digestive tract—specifically, your bowels. Constipation is more than just when your stool is hard and dry. It is also a difficulty in passing the said stool and when your stool is small and lumpy. The most common explanation of constipation in a Keto diet is the low fiber intake. The diet usually calls for a high intake of fats and protein to replace the carbohydrates you will not be eating. Fiber is primarily present in plants and fruits—it is in short supply when it comes to meat. People who have entered a state of Ketosis often experience constipation due to the lack of leafy vegetables and fruits in their diet. Fiber also works with water to form soft and easy-to-pass stool. The Ketogenic diet, however, promotes the release of water from the kidneys and cells.

Fats and proteins are overall more filling than carbohydrates—as a result, you will find yourself eating less. This is an ultimate benefit because you will stop yourself from overeating. However, it can also result in constipation because when you eat low amounts of highly satisfying food, digestion starts to slow down, and your bowels form fewer stools.

Yo-Yo Dieting

The Keto diet may sometimes result in yo-yo-ing because it is quite hard for people to stay on the restrictive diet for the long term. In a perfect world, it would be possible but this would not be possible over a lifetime. The problem with going back and forth is it can have negative effects on the body. People often find the diet hard to follow or stick to which leads it to becoming a fad and not taken as a serious lifestyle change.

Kidney and Heart Damage

Because the body is running low when it comes to electrolytes and fluid on top of the urination which has been increased, it may lead to a loss of electrolytes such as magnesium, sodium, and potassium. This would make you very prone to things like acute kidney injury.

Dehydration needs to be taken seriously as it may result in damage to the kidneys and lightheadedness. This may place the one on the diet at risk as well of cardiac arrhythmia considering the electrolytes which are required for normal heartbeats are not sufficient causing potential heart problems like irregularity. This is why it is important to take the

necessary supplements and foods to help prevent any health problems whilst on the diet.

Diarrhea

This is an ironic effect for some people as the Keto diet is supposed to ease such things as irritable bowel syndrome, but this is usually during the first few days. It can just be a result of the body trying to adjust to the macronutrient ratio changes as concerns protein and carb intake. In other scenarios, there are some who make the mistake of limiting the intake of fat along with the carbs and that means the protein intake is left to be the higher percentage which is harmful and could lead to diarrhea. Hence, the basis is to not skimp on the fats, as they are essential.

Muscle Cramps

The loss of minerals when you first start on the Keto diet can lead one to have muscle cramps, especially in the leg. In the same way with dealing with the other side effects mentioned, it would be advisable to drink a lot of water and eat salt which would go a long way in the prevention of cramps and reducing the loss of minerals to the body. It is also recommended that you take slow release magnesium tablets at the rate of 3 each day for a period of 20 days then you can reduce to one tablet a day for each day afterwards.

Nutritional Problems

The fear among most health experts is the high intakes of unhealthy fats may have a long-term negative effect. Weight loss, as such, may often time confuse the data for the short term. The reason is that when overweight people reduce their weight, regardless of how it happens they usually end up with better blood lipids and glucose levels. The Keto diet is also very restrictive against particular fruits, legumes, and grains which are originally thought of as the healthy choice. Without these foods, people that are on the diet can miss out on things like fiber, particular minerals, vitamins and phytochemicals which are only there in these foods. This has significant human health effects over the course of time like bone density reduction, and an increased risk of one suffering from chronic diseases.

Sleeping Problems

This affects a small number of people as the Keto diet is actually meant to improve the sleeping patterns. It could be as a result of their serotonin and insulin levels were low. In this case, you might try to have a snack before turning in for the night which has protein and some carbs in order to increase the levels of insulin. The other reason for bad sleep patterns could be the intake of food which is rich in histamines that cause anxiety and sleeplessness. This can be remedied by eating less, eggs, cheeses, and avocado which have histamines. They can instead be supplemented by starch free vegetables.

Pregnancy and Ketosis

When a woman is with child, the body goes through a number of changes. Even when a couple is trying to have a baby there will be a number of changes to the diet. As such, it may surprise you to know that Ketosis can actually be helpful for pregnancy. It has been recommended for women that have polycystic ovarian syndrome who have had issues with getting pregnant.

At the same time, just as a well-planned Keto diet would be safe for the average individual; it is also safe for those women trying to get pregnant especially if she was eating the standard American diet of high-carb foods before she went to the low-carb option. Now since it is helpful to use Ketosis to get pregnant the question becomes whether it is safe for someone to continue with Ketosis during the pregnancy.

There is a lot of misguiding information available through concerning Ketosis and pregnancy. When anyone refers to Ketosis not being a safe option during the term of pregnancy they are usually talking about studies on diabetic Ketoacidosis which is harmful and different as compared to Nutritional

Ketosis. There is a need to look at the differences. Diabetic Ketoacidosis is a dangerous metabolic state which is seen in people with diabetes where insulin or the diet would not be managed in the right manner. Diabetic Ketoacidosis pertains levels of ketones which are not naturally high and blood sugar levels that are three or more times as high as the norm. That would initiate a dangerous acid-based balance within the body. Ketoacidosis needs to be avoided in pregnant women.

Natural Scenarios of Ketosis in Women Who Are Pregnant

A lot of pregnant women suffer from morning sickness during the beginning stages of their pregnancy. Between that, low appetite, food aversion, and nausea, it is not uncommon for eating to be sporadic and usually in low amounts, especially during the early stages of the pregnancy. This will naturally happen—taking women in and out of Ketosis. Ketosis is natural as a part of being human. Between the time that you eat a meal and waking up in the morning, the body tends to be doing the fasting process, considering the first meal of the day is called "breakfast" for a reason. This is true for everyone including the ones that are pregnant. At the same time, the state of pregnancy could favor the Ketosis process. That is because the blood Ketone levels within women who are healthy and pregnant could, after a fast overnight, be much higher than that of women that are not with child.

Ketosis During the Late Stage of Pregnancy

It would seem then that Ketosis occurs on pregnant women a lot especially in the later stages. The fetus utilizes the ketones before and after the time of birth so as to make essential fats in the brain during development. Researchers claim even that fetuses may even make their ketones which would be part of the reason why Ketosis is more common in pregnant women during the third trimester. During the later stages of pregnancy, the metabolism of the woman also switches to the catabolic state which is the breaking down of molecules.

The Controversy When It Comes to the Keto Diet

Ketones in the urine of women who are pregnant tend to scare doctors into fearing for the life-threatening conditions. Still, the number of the primary care and OB/GYN physicians

It has become apparent though through some long-term observational studies that the unique physiological conditions which take place during pregnancy predict the future risk for the mothers and their children. As such, fostering a healthy pregnancy would be the essential thing for both the mother and her young one. The question then becomes the optimal diet for the woman and her specific conditions for the sake of her pregnancy. Into this vacuum of research, the doctors by default offer recommendations such as eating low fat, plenty of fruit veggies and grains. Some have even claimed that a woman who is doing a low-carb or Ketogenic diet is harming the baby.

The Low-Carb States and Pregnancy

There are a few case studies out there, one of which was a person who went through two high-carb filled pregnancies and a third pregnancy that was Keto based. The advantage that came with the latter one was quite clear according to her. She made the decision to switch to the Keto diet about 16 weeks into the pregnancy and the effects were brutal at first but after a day, the effects subsided. She claims that it is obvious that the body was meant to run on fat and protein so she cannot do carbs. She also said that her two previous pregnancies were wrought with issues such as high blood pressure, nausea, and infections as well as, bloating. In the Keto one, she says that blood pressure was normal and the weight gain was not obscene as she did not experience any bloating or swelling.

From this testimony, it would seem safe and perhaps even recommended for women to eat low amounts of carbs during pregnancy so long as they are still eating particular foods for the sake of proper nutrition. The fetuses need both ketones and glucose in order to grow which means the key, in this case, is a balance. The important thing to ensure is the mother had normal blood sugar levels and is getting a sufficient amount of calories.

Precautions

Even though Ketosis is safe and if it is done the right way, a lot of changes happen to the body of the women so extra precautions have to be taken during the time of pregnancy. The following are just a few tips that you need to keep in mind.

Do not have the objective of weight loss: The Keto diet may be the most effective diet plan for weight loss but for a lot of pregnant women, this would not be the optimal time to have it as a goal. No matter what way of eating is being followed, getting the right amount of calories and nutrition would be the most important thing.

Eat whole foods: speaking of nutrition, it is significant during the development of the fetus to eat whole foods. There are some carbs that are important for women who are pregnant to include within their diets such as seeds, nuts, legumes and fruits as well as, dairy.

Do not engage in intermittent fasting: Though intermittent fasting comes with a variety of benefits for the average individual, it would not be good during the pregnancy phase as the hunger cues do not come from dependency on carbs but what the baby needs so both the mother and the baby need to make sure they are getting the right amount of nutrients for their health.

Avoid eating refined sugars: the quality of carbs is something important to make sure that the diet is dense in nutrients and both the mother and the baby are getting the elements that they need in order to thrive.

Chapter 6

COMMON MISTAKES PEOPLE MAKE ON KETO

The Keto diet is highly beneficial to people; there are many success stories and it has become one of the most popular diets of this century. However, as popular as it may be, the Keto diet is not the easiest thing in the world. It requires you to take a keen focus on what you are doing and for many; it is a struggle because you will be completely changing your lifestyle. Your body is making internal changes which will cause you to do things differently.

Most people struggle to make the transition into Keto and when the body struggles, mistakes are made. While mistakes are not necessarily a big deal, in the Keto world they are a bad thing mentally and health wise. When you start on Keto, you usually expect to see results because others have seen remarkable results. When these things do not happen, it becomes very frustrating and will ultimately lead you into believing that Keto is not the diet for you. Before you can kick Keto to the curb, you should be open to the fact you may be making mistakes that are holding you back. Therefore, look out for the following common mistakes that people (and probably you) make on Keto.

#1 – The Wrong Fats

Since the minute people started getting into diet and exercise, the media and bad science have highly discouraged the consumption of any types of fat. All fatty foods were cast out for decades being proven to be unhealthy and not in any way helpful in weight loss. This advice is wrong because as the Keto diet has proven, fats can be good for weight loss and maintaining a healthy lifestyle. However, this does not mean that you should eat every fatty food you can find; not all fat is healthy. Not all fats are created equal, for Keto, you need to consume high-quality fats. The bad fats that people struggle with are the processed fats which are found in processed vegetable oils. Such fats have links to a variety of problems such as oxidation issues, inflammation, and adverse effects on vascular function.

The fats that you should be consuming are saturated fats; mono-saturated fats, polyunsaturated fats, and naturally occurring fats. Getting these types of fats is quite easy if you are looking to avoid all forms of trans-fats. You can find naturally occurring oils form avocadoes, coconuts, and olives. The good fats can also be found in butter, eggs, walnuts, and of course fish oils. Avoid fast food as much as possible because they are rich in unsaturated fats which are a gateway to problematic diseases such as high blood pressure, high levels of cholesterol which in turn leads to serious heart diseases.

#2 – Eating Too Much Protein

Eating too much protein is the mistake that tends to catch people completely off guard. Because you cannot eat carbohydrates and you cannot survive on fats alone, people increase their protein intake which is not bad unless it is done excessively. Growing up, it is common to hear that protein is good for you and it is best when it is consumed in control amounts. Many of us have faced rashes and breakouts when they consume too much protein. The issue with the Keto diet is that because your body is using fats as a fuel source, you will need a steady supply of protein to help maintain muscle mass. People go overboard with protein convincing themselves that they have a lot to make up for since they are not eating carbohydrates. Surprisingly, you will not need as much protein as you would expect to maintain your muscle mass. You see—when you consume more protein than your body actually needs, the body starts converting the protein into glucose, which then raises your blood sugar levels and takes you out of the state of Ketosis. In order to stop yourself from eating too much protein, focus instead on your macros. Your macros will prevent you from having anything in excess and you will only have what you need.

#3 - Too Little Water

When you are on a Keto diet, your body will instantly lose a lot of fluids. This means that you will need to stay hydrated as often as possible. For some reason, people seem to forget about water; this is extremely dangerous. When you restrict yourself of carbohydrates, several things happen to the body. One of these effects is that the levels of circulating blood-glucose and insulin fall drastically. Consider that many people eating a standard western diet have high levels of circulating insulin; high levels of insulin cause the kidneys to store more sodium which means that the kidneys will be retaining more fluids. Many people who start the diet complain of headaches which are caused by dehydration and an electrolyte imbalance. When you are not properly hydrated, your body will also store as much fat as possible which will be the opposite of what you are trying to achieve. This also means that your body will not be able to function properly; the heart will struggle to pump blood to the brain and that is what will cause you headaches.

You may not always enjoy drinking water but in order to do the Keto diet successfully, you will need to drink as much water as possible. The recommended amount of water is roughly a gallon a day; this is difficult to achieve but a few sips here and there through the day are bound to get you there. If you are going to add alcoholic drinks to your lifestyle, the amount should be more because alcohol dehydrates the body. You can also follow the general rule of 0.5 oz. to 1 oz. of every pound of body weight. In other words, just make sure you are drinking enough fluids, monitor what type of fluids you drink, and take your thirst seriously.

#4 – Focusing on the Food Alone

Keto diet is more than just about the food. You cannot just replace the bad foods that you consumed with Keto foods then expect to notice an immediate change. You have to change other parts of your lifestyle too if you want to achieve a healthy regime or weight loss depending on what your goal is. Of course, this is not easy to achieve and it is why most people make the mistake of simply focusing on food intake. If you focus on the food alone, you will not be able to achieve Ketosis. Because you will be eating high amounts of fat, the body will need to burn it off somehow. If you do not get an outlet to burn this fat such as working out or any other physical activity, the fat will not be burnt, you will not produce ketones, and you will never enter the state of Ketosis. Subtle changes such as walking around the block every day are sure to jog up your body into fat burning. You can increase this week after week or start an exercise regime to improve your lifestyle. Other small changes such as sitting less, walking more, doing daily jogs, and taking up yoga will be beneficial and will work together with the diet to give you the best results.

#5 – Obsessing Over Weight

One of the most common effects of the Keto diet is the weight loss. Even if you are not trying to lose weight, if you do the Keto diet properly you will definitely lose weight in a healthy way. It is very common in this century to see celebrities and even your friend post about the success they have had with Keto; posts of losing weight are the most common. The problem with focusing on these success stories is that it makes you directly drawn to the idea that all the progress is supposed to happen on the scale.

Unfortunately, everyone has a different body both on the outside and the inside and while you may be led to believe that progress is on the scale, you should know that it is not. Some people will drop weight almost immediately while for others it will take some time. Others will enter the state of Ketosis immediately while for others it will take weeks before they start producing ketones. The one thing that seems to change for people are the measurements; it is not surprising to hear that one has lost an inch or two in key areas of their bodies but it is ultimately very impressive. While you will want to keep track of how much weight you are losing for the sake of your health, you should not make it your ultimate measure of success. If you want to see real progress, you should take your measurements at least once a week. Measurement will help you to see the results that the scale will not show.

Chapter 7

Recipes & Meal Plans

When it comes to the beginning of the Keto diet or any other diets, there is something that everyone agrees on—having a plan before embarking on the objective. It is not wise to try and wing it with a Keto diet. No one has that kind of self-control, apparently, so all you will be doing is lying to yourself about the abilities of your mind, albeit slowly sinking into the abyss that is the carb diet once more. The trouble with backsliding on a diet is that it will prove to you that you do not have what it takes to seriously eat at your confidence. The odds of you trying to go on a similar diet during the foreseeable future would be absolutely minimal or zero. Hence, you need a plan to guide yourself by. Set a start date, and then prepare through reorganizing the pantry or through working out some of your meal and snack options. You can even purchase appropriate foods and the diet supplements that you would need in advance to be proactive.

It has been proven that the biggest reason that people have a hard time sticking by the Keto diet they embarked on, is that they do not have sufficient interesting foods that they can go to at any time. In this case, regardless of all the good intentions in the world, you will still find that high-carb addictive foods will win. If you did not buy the food at the store that fits the regulations that have been set, then it will not be an easy option in the fridge if you need it. The other thing is that it is crucial to make sure the diet is set ahead of time because the foods that are available to be chosen are limited.

At the same time, you would be recommended to consult a physician in order to make them aware you are starting a diet, which is going to change the way your body tends to metabolize food into energy. It would also be advisable that you go in to check the most recent blood-work levels when it comes to things such as vitamin D, cholesterol and other health indicators — as these are liable to change when one is undergoing the Keto diet. The reason is that for some individuals, a Keto diet that is prolonged may result in a nutritional deficiency or high levels of cholesterol.

The majority of experts are going to say that the Keto diet was not meant to be a permanent lifestyle option. The one thing that is admired concerning the diet and the related meal plans would be that tracking of the food is actually optional. There is no requirement set to meticulously go through the calories, which would be the case when it comes to other diets. Because one is increasing their intake of both fat and protein, there is a higher likelihood to be satiated and have the energy for the whole day — and that causes the individual to eat at a lesser rate. Now, that is not to say that food tracking when it comes to the Keto diet is out of the question. There are some that could find the calorie counting as something beneficial in order to be aware of what they are consuming, but it is not mandatory when you are on the Keto diet. There should not be a need for you to become too stressed concerning meeting the particular caloric objectives, particularly if losing weight is not the specific objective in this case.

One of the areas where food tracking would be taken as helpful, though, is when making sure that the person is hitting the particular high ratios of macronutrients when it comes to protein, carbs, and fat.

The current version of the Keto diet apparently derives that 70 percent of the healthy calories would come from fats, 20 would be from the proteins, and the rest would be from carbohydrates. In the ideal setting, each meal and even snacks should have this ratio concerning the macronutrients, though research is showing that you would still be able to get good results even if each meal deviates slightly from this ratio for as long as the person does not exceed 50 grams of carbs in a particular setting. Hence, to achieve the ratios without first having a preset meal plan from the dietician or the physician, there would have to be a certain amount of tracking meals — but once you get the hang of things, it would not be needed as much anymore. Similarly, the frequency of the meals should also be up to the preference of a person. There are recommendations of up to four servings a day with a few Keto-oriented snacks in between, and this ensures that you would be getting a mix of protein and fat every day so as to keep you satisfied and energized. You should just listen to what the body needs and tune in to when it is truly hungry — as opposed to when it just wants to snack. If you find that eating smaller meals of six during the entire day is what works for you, then proceed, provided that you do not go above the quota of 50 grams of carbs every day, as overfeeding on the Keto diet would also be counter-productive for obvious purposes.

How Do Meal Plans Work?

The meal plan has 4 meals every day with recipes that would otherwise be filling, and every meal is distributed according to an equal manner in calories in order to give the maximum amount of satisfaction.

In order for one to make up for the less amount of consumption, the four meals equally split the entire calories so that it becomes 400 calories for every meal—and in a day, there would be an intake of 1200 to 1600 calories. Each meal becomes fulfilling, and eating these four in a day would consume less time as opposed to when you have 6 meals. Within the complete Keto diet, only 5 percent of the calories come from the carbs, 20 percent from the protein, and the remaining percentage from healthy fats. This is to say that Keto-adaptation is allowed from the current eating lifestyle. Each meal would come with 5 net grams or less.

How to Find the Daily Need?

There is a particular calorie need for every individual. Yours would depend upon things like size, fitness, and daily activities as well. When you are setting a healthy Keto meal plan, the first thing to do would be to calculate the equilibrium for the calories. That is to say the number of calories that are needed each day to maintain the same weight. Once you become aware of the calorie equilibrium, then you will become able to adjust the daily calories upwards or downwards so as to meet the objectives which you have set. If the goal is a loss of weight, then the recommendation would be eating 3 to 5 hundred calories less than the standard equilibrium every day. Take note, though that this should not be lower than 1200 calories every day. That would then lead to a steady rate of weight loss in a healthy manner. On the other hand, if you were of the objective to gain muscle, then you could begin by adding the same proportion of about three to five hundred calories every day more than your equilibrium — and see the results. If the result is that you are putting on fat as opposed to muscle mass, then you may opt to decrease the calories slightly.

The Keto meal plan is simple and quick to prepare an optimize if the right macro ratios are already calculated for you such that all you would need to do would be making your meals. Each of the meals that are in the plan takes about 25 minutes or less. The calories also seem to add up to 1600 calories in total from four meals if set in a table format and added up.

Snack Recipes for the Keto Diet

Here are some practical recipes to kickstart your keto diet:

Cheesy Zucchini

Time needed: 15 minutes

Servings: 2

Here is a recipe for a cheesy, fulfilling side dish. It is simple and quick, yet delicious enough to serve with every meal if you want. Even kids will love this zucchini because of the addition of all the cheesy goodness. Your family will not even miss your old macaroni and cheese. Enjoy this low carb recipe with almost any main course. It is a perfect pairing to add just a bit more fats and protein to the meal.

This is especially ideal for **Standard/Targeted Ketogenic Diet.**

Ingredients:

- shredded cheddar cheese, organic, full-fat – 1 cup
- water – .5 cup
- salt – 1 tea spoon
- ghee, organic, grass-fed – 1 tea spoon
- heavy cream, organic, full-fat – 2 tea spoon
- zucchini, organic – 1

1. Wash the zucchini and slice it into circular slices.
2. Boil the water with the zucchini slices and the salt, stirring occasionally.
3. Reduce the heat to low. Stir in the cream, the butter, and the cheese, and cook the combination until it is well incorporated.
4. Remove the dish from the heat and serve.

Macros:

- 315 calories
- 7-gram protein
- 9-gram fat
- 1-gram net carbs

Green Bean Stir Fry

Time needed: 15 minutes

Servings: 4

This Asian inspired side dish is savory and delicious. It pairs well with salmon, chicken, pork, or beef. Try this out, and it is guaranteed to become a fast favorite, due to the flavors and the ease of preparation. Always great to eat immediately, this also will be an awesome option for meal prep sides. For a side dish, this recipe is relatively high in fat, so it will aid you in feeling fuller longer, which makes it great for evening meals.

This is especially ideal for **High-Protein Ketogenic Diet.**

Ingredients:

- salt – 1 tea spoon
- ghee, grass-fed – 1 tea spoon
- yellow onion, organic, large – .5
- minced garlic, organic – 2 tea spoons
- green beans, organic, fresh – 1 pound

1. Wash and trim the green beans. Cut them into 2-inch-long strips.
2. Peel and slice the onion to make 2-inch strips.
3. Melt the ghee in a wok or frying pan over high heat.
4. Stir fry the garlic and the onion for one minute.
5. Add the green beans, and cook them for two minutes, stirring often.
6. Remove the stir-fry from the heat, sprinkle on the salt over the top, and serve.

Macros:

- 182 calories
- 9 grams protein
- 12 grams fat
- 0 grams of net carbs

Keto Egg Muffins

Serves 3

This is especially ideal for **Standard/Targeted Ketogenic Diet.**

Ingredients

- Quarter cup red onion chopped
- One cup mixed greens
- 8 egg yolks
- 1/3 cup bacon crumbled
- One and a half cup cheddar cheese
- Half a teaspoon of garlic salt
- Four cherry tomatoes

Instructions

1. Separate the yolks from the whites in a big mixing bowl. Discard the whites.
2. Wash and chop the greens, onion, and tomatoes—then add to the mixture of the yolk.

3. Add cheese, unsweetened almond milk, bacon, and salt to the mixing bowl with the veggies.
4. Grease the muffin tin with oil, and then proceed to pour a quarter cup and a tablespoon of the egg mixture into the muffin slows that would yield about six of them.
5. Pop the tray into the oven for a time of about 12 minutes or to the point that the edges become toasty brown.
6. Serve after a few minutes.

Parmesan and Chive Mashed Cauliflower

Time needed: 15 minutes

Servings: 4

You will never miss mashed potatoes again. This cauliflower version is so savory; you won't even miss carbs. Enjoy this smooth and creamy side dish with everything from pork medallions to steaks. You can add full-fat butter or grass-fed ghee if needed to allow the recipe to contain higher levels of fat, and add an irresistible buttery flavor.

This is especially ideal for **Cyclical Ketogenic Diet.**

Ingredients:

- chives, organic, fresh, chopped – .25 cups
- parmesan cheese, organic, fresh, full-fat, grated – .25 cups
- chicken broth, organic – 2 cups
- cauliflower, organic – 2 small heads, chopped

1. Boil the cauliflower and the chicken broth for 10 minutes.
2. Drain the cauliflower and blend it in a blender until it is smooth.
3. Stir in the parmesan cheese and the chives. Add salt and black pepper to taste.
4. The dish is ready to serve.

Macros:

- 168 calories
- 3-gram protein
- 2-gram fat
- 4 grams of net carbs.

Pepperoni Pizza Bites

Serves 1

This is especially ideal for **Standard/Targeted Ketogenic Diet.**

Ingredients

- 2 tablespoons of pizza sauce
- 3 oz. of mozzarella
- 1 tablespoon of fresh oregano
- 6 slices of sandwich sliced pepperoni

Instructions

1. Preheat the oven to a level of 200 degrees Celsius. Snip a half-inch cuts around the edges of each slice of pepperoni — leaving the center uncut.
2. Press each of the pepperoni slices down into the regular-sized muffin pans. Bake the slices for a time of five minutes up to the point the edges are still crisp, though they are bright red. Remove them from the oven, and then

let the slices become cool in pans so that they become hard.
3. As the pepperoni cups are still cooking, you can dice the fresh oregano.
4. So as to remove the excess oil after the bites have been cooked, place them on a towel for a period of 10 minutes the way you would sausages.
5. Wipe the grease from the muffin pan with a paper towel, and then return the cups to the pan. Place a tablespoon of pizza sauce and half an oz. of mozzarella in every cup—then sprinkle with oregano.
6. You can place the bites back within the oven for a time of a few minutes of up to the time that the cheese starts to melt.
7. Allow for the bites to begin cooling down for a time of five minutes.

Spicy Riced Cauliflower

Time needed: 10 minutes

Servings: 4

Give your cauliflower a kick with this Mexican inspired flavor. Pair this side with salads or poultry. If pairing with a salad, be sure to include a full-fat dressing, nuts, seeds, or avocado to up the fat intake from the meal. This recipe makes four servings, so you can use it as a side in meal preps if you wish, as well. Just store any extras in the refrigerator for up to five days.

This is especially ideal for **Cyclical Ketogenic Diet.**

Ingredients:

- salt – to taste
- chili powder – .25 tea spoon
- garlic powder, organic – 1 tea spoon
- bone broth, organic – .25 cup
- tomato sauce, organic – .5 cups
- olive oil, extra virgin, organic – 1 tea spoon
- cauliflower rice, organic – 20 oz. freezer bag

1. Heat the olive oil in a frying pan over high heat.
2. Add the cauliflower rice to the frying pan.
3. In a bowl, combine the bone broth, the tomato sauce, the chili powder, and the garlic powder.
4. Pour the mix into the frying pan with the cauliflower and mix it in well.
5. Cook the combination for one minute longer, and then remove it from the heat source.
6. Add salt to taste and serve.

Macros:

- 190 calories
- 1-gram protein
- 1-gram fat
- 3 grams of net carbs

Breakfast Recipes

Blueberry Keto Protein Smoothie

Time needed: 5 minutes

Servings: 1

This fruity smoothie can be a quick breakfast on the go or even just a snack. With the addition of a high-quality protein powder (grass-fed protein powders are best), this recipe is perfect for a delicious post-workout meal. For variance, just switch out the type of berries used. Strawberries, raspberries, and blackberries work well too. You could even throw in a handful of mixed berries to create a more complex flavor. The protein and fat contained within this smoothie will allow you to feel full for much longer than a typical fruit smoothie would. If you choose to use frozen berries, there is no need to thaw them, as they will provide a bit of iciness and thickness to the smoothie that will make you feel like you are having a milkshake for breakfast.

This is especially ideal for a **High-Protein Ketogenic Diet.**

Ingredients:

- protein powder, grass-fed, organic – 1 scoop
- extra virgin olive oil, organic – 1 tea spoon
- vanilla extract, organic – 1 tea spoon
- blueberries, organic, fresh or frozen – .25 cup
- coconut milk, organic – 1 cup

- Place all of the listed ingredients in a blender and mix them until you reach a desired smooth texture.

Macros:

- 343 calories
- 31 grams protein
- 21 grams fat
- 3 grams of net carbs

Eggs and Vegetables Fried in Coconut Oil

Ingredients

- Carrots
- Cauliflower
- Broccoli
- Green beans
- Spices
- Spinach

Instructions

1. Add coconut oil to the frying pan and heat it.
2. Add vegetables. Use a frozen mix and let it thaw during the heat for some time.
3. Add eggs.
4. Add the spices. Use a spice mix, although salt and pepper work effectively.
5. Add spinach.
6. Stir fry up to the point it is ready.

Egg and Bacon Scramble

Time needed: 15 minutes

Servings: 1

Combine the all-time breakfast favorites of eggs and bacon in this scrumptious scramble. Start your day off right with a quick and creative take on this classic breakfast that will leave you feeling full all morning. This recipe has higher amounts of fat and protein while remaining low in carbs. This will leave you satiated while allowing your body to run on the fats.

This is especially ideal for the **Standard/Targeted Ketogenic Diet.**

Ingredients:

- eggs, whole, organic, cage-free – 2
- bacon, chopped, natural, full-fat, uncured – 2 slices
- parsley, organic, chopped, – 1 ounce
- black pepper and salt

1. In a pan or skillet, fry the chopped bacon pieces over medium to high heat.

2. Add the eggs and the parsley to the pan.
3. Scramble all of the ingredients together.
4. Add black pepper and salt to suit your taste.

Macros:

- 136 calories
- 8 grams protein
- 11 grams of fat
- 1 gram net carbs.

Egg, Bacon, and Avocado Tacos

Time needed: 15 minutes

Servings: 2

These breakfast tacos will give you a balanced, filling start to your day. The eggs are used as the taco shell, in an innovative way to cut out unnecessary carbs and utilize more eggs in your diet. Serve these tacos immediately or make them ahead as meal prep. Just reheat them in the microwave for 45 seconds, and your breakfast will be ready. This recipe is great for Taco Tuesday and any other day as well! The eggs provide protein, and the avocado and ghee will give you plenty of fat. This meal will leave you filled with energy and feeling full.

This is especially ideal for the **Standard/Targeted Ketogenic Diet.**

Ingredients:

- bacon, uncured, natural – 2 slices
- romaine lettuce, organic – .25 cup
- pink Himalayan salt – .25 of a tea spoon
- avocado, organic – 1
- ghee, organic, grass-fed – 1 tea spoon

➢ eggs, organic, cage-free – 2

1. In order to make the taco "shells," melt one tablespoon of ghee in a small skillet over medium-high heat.
2. In the center of the skillet, crack one egg, making sure that the yolk is broken.
3. Cook the egg on both sides until it is completely solid.
4. Remove the egg from the pan and set it aside for later.
5. With the second egg, repeat steps one through four to make a second taco shell.
6. Smash the avocado in a small bowl with a fork.
7. Spread one half of the mashed avocado on each egg taco shell.
8. Place one half of the romaine lettuce on each taco.
9. Add one bacon slice on each shell.
10. Fold the shells in half and enjoy your meal.

Macros:

- 387 calories
- 11 grams protein
- 35 grams fat
- 4 grams of net carbs

Keto Porridge

Time needed: 10 minutes

Servings: 1

With fewer carbs than other hot cereals, this Keto porridge can meet and surpass your cravings on a cold winter morning. This porridge is filling, cozy, and ready just as quickly as any traditional oatmeal. There is no need to add carbs to your diet with oatmeal, cream of wheat, or grits. Instead, use this recipe to give you the feeling of having a warm bowl of porridge. It is high in fat to keep you fulfilled and provide sustained energy to start your day off well.

This is especially ideal for the **Standard/Targeted Ketogenic Diet.**

Ingredients:

- salt – 1 tea spoon
- coconut milk, organic – 2 tea spoons
- coconut flour, organic – 1 tea spoon
- egg, whole, organic, cage-free – 1
- ghee, organic, grass-fed – 1 ounce
- berries, organic, fresh or frozen

1. In a nonstick saucepan, add all of the ingredients, with the exception of the berries and the coconut milk.
2. Stirring constantly, mix the ingredients well over low heat.
3. Add the coconut milk and stir.
4. Remove the pan from the heat and spoon the porridge into a bowl.
5. Serve with fresh or thawed frozen berries as a garnish.

Macros:

- 486 calories
- 8 grams protein
- 49 grams fat
- 4 grams of net carbs

Mushroom Omelet

Time needed: 15 minutes

Servings: 1

This mushroom omelet is so delicious you will end up wanting to eat it for lunches and dinners as well! It is an easy and filling way to start your day with all of your favorite savory flavors. Mushrooms, cheese, and onion pack plenty of flavors. The high amount of fat and the protein that this recipe contains will allow you to feel fully content, and provide the energy and mental clarity needed to make it through your morning.

This is especially ideal for **High-Protein Ketogenic Diet.**

Ingredients:

- black pepper and salt
- mushrooms, organic, fresh, sliced – 3
- yellow onion, organic, fresh, diced – .25 tea spoon
- shredded cheddar cheese, organic, full-fat – 1 ounce

- full-fat butter or ghee, organic, grass-fed – 1 ounce
- eggs, whole, organic, cage-free – 3

1. Mix all of the eggs into a bowl while adding a pinch of each black pepper and salt.
2. In a frying pan, melt the butter over medium heat.
3. Pour in the mixture of eggs.
4. As the bottom of the omelet begins to cook, put the sliced mushrooms, cheese, and diced onion on top, covering one half of the omelet.
5. Fold the omelet in half and continue cooking it. You will know the omelet is finished when it is a light golden brown in color.

Macros:

- 272 calories
- 15-gram protein
- 22-gram fat
- 1-gram net carbs

Lunch Recipes

Jar Salad

Time needed: 10 minutes

Servings: 1

This is perfect for a delicious and healthy lunch on the go. It is great to pack up and take to work or school. A plethora of beautiful colors and flavors delight all the senses as you enjoy this salad. The dressing will provide the majority of the fat in this recipe, so do not feel the need to skimp on it. With the addition of protein, this salad will be quite filling. The recipe may be varied by adding nuts or cheese, or by changing up the source of protein. Feel free to make additions such as cabbage or to swap a particular vegetable for something you like better. The possibilities are endless.

This is especially ideal for **High-Protein Ketogenic Diet.**

Ingredients:

- mayonnaise, organic, full-fat, or olive oil, organic – 4 tea spoons
- scallions, organic, fresh, chopped – 1 tea spoon
- cucumber, organic, sliced – .25 cup
- red bell pepper, organic, sliced – .25 cup
- cherry tomatoes, organic, halved – .25 cup
- leafy greens of your choice, organic (spinach, kale, arugula, etc.) – .5 cup
- rotisserie chicken, smoked salmon, or boiled egg – 4 ounces

1. Chop the vegetables into small slices or cubes, based on your preference.
2. Layer the ingredients in a mason jar. Leafy greens go on the bottom, with scallions next, followed by the red bell peppers, then cucumbers and tomatoes. The top and final layer will be the protein source of your choice.
3. Package the olive oil or mayonnaise separately from the salad to use as dressing.

The addition of the dressing before you are ready to eat will cause the salad to be soggy.

Macros:

- 247 calories
- 25-gram protein
- 16-gram fat
- .5-gram net carbs

Keto Burgers

Time needed: 15 minutes

Servings: 3

Nothing beats a classic juicy burger on a warm summer evening. Now you can make a delicious burger with only a few simple ingredients. Olive oil or ghee can be used to create extra juiciness. Thanks to the added ghee or olive oil, each burger patty comes in at a whopping 40 grams of fat. Combined with protein provided by this meal, it is a delicious way to maintain a feeling of satisfaction. Wrap each burger patty up in a soft butter lettuce leaf to cut the use of any unnecessary carbs in the form of a hamburger bun. Make extra and store them in the freezer to reheat later! They also work well for meal prep, staying good in the refrigerator for up to three days.

This is especially ideal for **Standard/Targeted Ketogenic Diet.**

Ingredients:

- black pepper and salt – .5 tea spoon each
- Worcestershire sauce – 1 tea spoon

- ➢ ground beef, organic, grass-fed – 1 pound
- ➢ olive oil, extra virgin, organic, or ghee, organic, grass-fed – 2 tea spoons
- ➢ butter lettuce, organic – 3 large leaves

1. Preheat the grill or a skillet to medium-high heat.
2. Use your hands to distribute the Worcestershire sauce, pepper, salt, and your choice of olive oil or ghee evenly through the ground beef as you break the meat up.
3. Form the meat into three patties. This is done by rolling them into balls, flattening them, and then creating a divot with a thumbprint in the center of each burger patty. The divets will help the patties maintain their uniform shape while cooking, instead of rising in the middle.
4. Cook or grill the patties to your personal favorite "doneness."
5. Serve up the cooked patties in the butter lettuce leaves with your favorite condiments and additions. Just remember to track any

added carbs and add them to the total that have been listed for this recipe.

Macros:

- 479 calories
- 26 grams protein
- 40 grams fat
- 0 grams of net carbs

Keto Chicken Nuggets

Time needed: 15 minutes

Servings: 6

This Keto version tastes just like traditional chicken nuggets. They are super quick to make, as they use pre-cooked chicken. The use of precooked meat gives them a soft texture that is truly satisfying. This recipe is great for family meals and can also be prepped ahead of time. The chicken nuggets can be stored in the freezer and reheated later. The recipe calls for precooked chicken meat, so you can provide this meat in a few ways. You can use part of a rotisserie chicken, or use any leftovers you may have from a lunch or dinner. This is a great way to not let leftovers go to waste, as you can whip these up with any leftover chicken from a previous recipe, and have the basis of a full meal.

This is especially ideal for **High-Protein Ketogenic Diet or Cyclical Ketogenic Diet.**

Ingredients:

- garlic powder – 1 tea spoon
- almond flour, organic – .25 cups

- egg, organic, cage-free – 1 whole
- cream cheese, organic, full-fat – 8 ounces
- chicken, organic, free range, cooked – 2 cups

1. With an electric mixer, shred the chicken into small pieces. This will work most easily if the chicken meat is warm. You can use rotisserie chicken or leftover chicken from another recipe.
2. Mix in the rest of the ingredients listed.
3. Once everything is thoroughly combined, place a spoonful of the chicken mixture on a baking sheet that is covered with parchment paper. Flatten the meat scoops to create the shape of traditional chicken nuggets.
4. Bake for 12-13 minutes at 350 degrees. You will know that the chicken nuggets are finished when the nuggets are firm and a light golden brown in color.

Macros:

- 243 calories
- 18 grams protein
- 17 grams fat
- 2 grams of net carbs

Low-Carb Keto Lasagna

This is especially ideal for **Standard/Targeted Ketogenic Diet.**

Ingredients

- 1 tea spoon of butter, coconut oil, or even lard
- ½ spicy Italian sausage
- 2 tea spoons of coconut flour
- 15 oz. ricotta cheese
- Medium to large whole egg
- 1 ½ teaspoon of salt
- ½ teaspoon of pepper
- 1/3 cup parmesan cheese
- A large clove garlic
- 4 large zucchini's
- 1 ½ mozzarella cheese

Instructions

1. Slice the zucchini then sprinkle with sea salt. Put the salted zucchini on a paper towel for a time of 30 minutes. Once the time is up, wring the zucchini noodles with a paper towel, and extract moisture.

2. Heat the tablespoon of butter or fat depending on your preference in a large skillet using medium level heating. Crumble and brown the Italian sausage.
3. Preheat the oven to a level of 375 degrees, and then coat the baking dish with butter.
4. Add the ricotta cheese, 2 tea spoons of parmesan cheese, 1 egg, coconut flour, garlic, salt, and pepper to a small bowl and then mix them. Set this aside, and then add Italian seasoning and red pepper to a jar of marinara and stir.
5. Add a layer of sliced zucchini to the bottom of the dish. Spread 14 cups of cheese over the zucchini, sprinkle with ¼ of the sausage and then add a layer. Repeat the process over three or four times up to the point the ingredients are done.
6. Cover using the foil, and bake for a time of 20 minutes.

Salmon and Asparagus

Time needed: 15 minutes

Servings: 2

Cook your whole dinner all in one frying pan. This recipe is great for families (just double the recipe), for a single meal, or for meal prep. This meal is everything you can ask for: delicious, fast, and healthy. The fat and protein from these ingredients will work well to keep you satiated long after eating. In Order not to become bored with this meal, just swap the salmon for dark meat chicken, or switch out the asparagus for broccoli. This is a classic recipe you can keep coming back to, while still providing a variance of flavors.

This is especially ideal for a **High-Protein Ketogenic Diet.**

Ingredients:

- black pepper and salt – to taste
- salmon, wild-sourced – 9 oz.
- ghee, organic, grass-fed – 3 ounces
- asparagus, organic, fresh – 8 oz.

1. Clean and trim the asparagus spears.
2. Melt the ghee in a large frying pan over medium heat.
3. For 3 to 5 minutes, fry the asparagus, and then move it all to one side of the pan.
4. Use the other half of the pan to fry the salmon for 2 minutes on each side. You can add a little bit more ghee if needed for the salmon to cook.
5. Season the salmon with black pepper and salt to taste and serve.

Macros:

- 512 calories
- 40-gram protein
- 30-gram fat
- 1-gram net carbs

Dinner Recipes

Broccoli Parmesan Soup

Time needed: 15 minutes

Servings: 6

There is nothing better than a bowl of hot soup on a chilly day. Try this filling and flavorful recipe. This is a soup that cooks up nicely for the whole family or to be used for meal prep. Leftovers can be stored in the freezer. This recipe alone does not contain a lot of fat, so be sure to pair it with something such as salmon or avocado to sustain enough energy from the meal that you will feel satisfied.

This is especially ideal for **High-Protein Ketogenic Diet or Cyclical Ketogenic Diet.**

Ingredients:

- lemon juice, organic, fresh – 2 T
- parmesan cheese, organic, full-fat, fresh – .75 cups
- water – 4 cups
- almond milk, organic, unsweetened – 2 cups

- broccoli florets, organic, fresh – 3 pounds

1. Place the broccoli in a large pot with the water. Cover with a lid and boil for 10 minutes.
2. Keep one cup of the cooking liquid from the broccoli and drain the rest.
3. Place one half of the broccoli in a blender, along with the reserved cooking liquid and the almond milk. Mix the ingredients until smooth, and return them to the pot with the remaining broccoli.
4. After adding lemon juice and cheese, cook the mixture for two more minutes. Remove the soup from the heat source and serve it while it still warm.

Macros:

- 85 calories
- 7-gram protein
- 3-gram fat
- 6 grams of net carbs

Parmesan Chicken in White Sauce

This is especially ideal for a High-Protein Ketogenic Diet.

Ingredients

- 2 teaspoons of olive oil
- 1 cup of cream
- 1 teaspoon of garlic powder
- 1 teaspoon of Italian seasoning
- ½ cup of chicken broth
- 1 ½ pounds of skinless boneless chicken breasts
- 1 cup of spinach
- ½ cup sun-dried tomatoes
- ½ cup parmesan cheese

Instructions

1. In a large skillet, add olive oil, and then cook the chicken with the use of medium heat for a few minutes till it browns on either side. Remove the chicken, and then set it aside.
2. Add the garlic powder, cream, parmesan cheese, Italian seasoning, and chicken broth.

Whisk when the mixture is in medium heat till it begins to thicken. Add sundried tomatoes and spinach, and then let it start to simmer to the point that the spinach begins to wilt. Add the chicken breasts to the pan, and then mix for a few minutes then serve.

Tomato Basil Keto Soup

Time needed: 15 minutes

Servings: 6

This is another super easy soup recipe to fill you up on cool evenings. Reminiscent of childhood, but healthy for you too. Fresh tomatoes lend an irresistible flavor, while cream cheese gives it a pleasing texture. Use this recipe all year long by serving it chilled like a gazpacho on warmer days as well. The levels of fat and protein in this recipe allow the sop to stand alone as a meal to be used as an appetizer or a side.

This is especially ideal for a **Standard/Targeted Ketogenic Diet.**

Ingredients:

- black pepper and salt to taste
- stevia – 1 tea spoon
- basil leaves, organic, fresh – .5 cup
- cream cheese, organic, full-fat – 8 ounces
- ghee, organic, grass-fed – 2 tea spoons
- tomatoes, organic, fresh – 6 large

1. Place the tomatoes into a blender and mix until they form a puree.
2. In a large pot, place the tomato puree over medium-high heat.
3. Add the cream cheese and the ghee to the tomato puree as it begins to cook. Continue cooking until the cheese and ghee are melted and well incorporated.

Macros:

- 287 calories
- 3 grams protein
- 28 grams fat
- 6 grams of net carbs

Zoodles

Time needed: 5 minutes

Servings: 2

Zoodles are simply zucchini in the shape of noodles. They will allow you to enjoy all of your favorite pasta recipes without the carbs. These "noodles" are low in calories and carbs, yet they will taste just as delicious as any other noodle you could try. Plus, they can be made very quickly, ready to serve in minutes, or as a part of meal prep. You will want to ensure that the sauces you choose to use have high amounts of fat and protein to make up most of the energy from this meal, as zucchini alone is not high in either.

This is ideal for a **High-Protein Ketogenic Diet or a Cyclical Ketogenic Diet.**

Ingredients:

- zucchini, organic – 4

1. If you have access to a spiralizer, use it to create noodles of zucchini. If you do not own

a spiralizer, this recipe is still very simple. Just slice the zucchini into long thin strips. You may also wish to use a cheese and vegetable grater to get the desired noodle effect.
2. Serve the zoodles as they are, or let them boil for two minutes in a pan of water to warm and soften them up a bit. Alternately, you may wish to sauté them in a bit of olive oil or ghee for a minute or two to give them a little crispness.
3. Serve the zoodles in place of the traditional noodles in your favorite pasta dishes.

Macros:

- 65 calories
- 5-gram protein
- 1-gram fat
- 4 grams of net carbs

www.ingramcontent.com/pod-product-compliance
Lightning Source LLC
Chambersburg PA
CBHW020256030426
42336CB00010B/791